Diabetes is a Choice

By

Gary L Moore

CONTENTS

FOREWORD

American Journal of Health Promotion: Facing the Facelessness of Public Health: Dr. David Katz director of Yale Griffin prevention research center wrote:

"We have known since 1993 at least, when "Actual Causes of Death in the United States" was published in the Journal of the American Medical Association, that the leading causes of both premature death and persistent misery in our society are chronic disease that are, in turn, attributable to the use of our feet (physical activity), forks (dietary pattern), and fingers (cigarette smoking). Feet, forks, and fingers are the master levels of medical destiny for not just thousands or tens of thousands of people on any one occasion but the medical destiny of millions of Americans year after year.

We as doctors have known but we have not managed to care. At least not care deeply enough to turn what we know into what we routinely do. Were we to do so, we could eliminate 80% of all heart disease and strokes, 90% of all diabetes, and as much as 60% of all cancer.

But saving millions of lives is just a number. He asked doctors to forget the bland statistics of public health and to ask yourself if you love someone who has suffered a heart attack, stroke, cancer, or diabetes. You are exceptional if you do not.

Now imagine their faces, whisper their names, recall what it felt like to get the news, and while at it, imagine the faces of other readers like you and me imagining beloved faces.

Now imagine if 8 of 10 of us wistfully reflecting on intimate love and loss, on personal anguish, never got that dreadful news because it never happened. Mom did not get cancer; dad did not have a heart attack; grandpa did not have a stroke; sister, brother, aunt, and uncle did not lose a limb or kidney or eyes to diabetes. We are all intimately linked in a world of a network of personal tragedy.

Which leads to what he asking the doctors to do about it: put a face on public health every chance you get. When talking about heart disease and its prevention, or cancer, or diabetes, ask your audience to see in their mind's eye the face of a loved one affected by that condition. Then ask them to imagine that loved one as beneficiary among the 80% who need never have succumbed if what we knew were what we do. Evoke the mind's eye then bring a tear to it."

I'm not a doctor but a doctor did not cure my atherosclerosis in fact the statins prescribed gave me rhabdomyolysis where your muscles break down so rapidly your urine starts looking like brown Kool-Aid as you literally start peeing your muscles down the toilet. Then your kidneys fail, and you die. Only about 1 in 6 or 7 million suffers enough muscle damage to kill them lucky me and to add to my dilemma I was diagnosed with diabetes about 1 out of 200 people on statins become diabetic.

When I graduated college my philosophy on health was exercise before work every day, don't eat junk food never drink alone or before 5 pm. Since heart disease is the number one killer in the western world and statins are the prescribed treatment, I searched for an alternative and discovered the work of Nathan Pritikin who reversed his heart disease in the 1950s and he explained entire cultures 100's of millions of people never get heart disease, diabetes, colon, breast, prostate, cancer, glaucoma, arthritis, cataracts, gallstones, and hypertension, evidently western diseases. I didn't want any of those diseases or anyone for that matter to suffer from these preventable chronic diseases so my avocation became researching research. Then I wanted to share this information with you! Because your life's worth it and you can become a role model for your family and friends.

The Diabetes epidemic and its' association with other diseases. are really frightening by midcentury 1 out of 3 Americans will be diabetic but the real trend is even higher. Over a hundred million diabetics will make our country insolvent according to United Health this one preventable disease will cost three and half trillion dollars a year. In essence our collective weight is going to collapse our country. How much avoidable misery does three and half trillion dollars represent.

The British National Health Service designates individuals on the diabetic register who are willing to do whatever it takes to reverse this hideous disease as "Health Motivated." Shouldn't we all be health motivated? I mistakenly thought I was!

In a 1979 report to the American people, the Surgeon General admonished us, "You, the individual, can do more for your own health and well-being than any doctor, any hospital, any drug, any exotic medical advice."

Caution to The Reader: If you are taking any medication, do not make dietary changes without the assistance of a physician.

3

It is even more important to consult with a knowledgeable physician who is familiar with the medication reduction needed as a result of aggressive dietary modifications. Do not underestimate how effective this program is because without medication reductions, a serious hypoglycemic reaction could occur from taking too much medication.

Many physicians, not realizing how effective this diet style is, may be hesitant to taper medications sufficiently. Make sure you warn your physician about this and follow your blood sugar carefully the first few weeks after beginning this plan. If you are on high blood pressure this may also lower your blood pressure too much, so be sure to watch that and discuss any changes with your physician.

I was on no medications to treat my diabetes but I have friends Type II diabetics for years on insulin off insulin in the first 10 days after going on the High Nutrient Dense Diet recommended and others' on medication cut their medication in half and off all medication in 3 to 6 months. This is serious get physician's assistance in reducing your medication that are knowledgeable.

Americans rather than taking an honest look at what causes diabetes, Americans are still looking for a magical, effortless cure for it -a gimmick, drug, or surgery. The only answer is living a healthy lifestyle focused on excellent nutrition along with adequate activity and exercise. When you live this way, the benefits will overwhelm genetics and allow even those people with a genetic predisposition to weight gain and diabetes to achieve a healthy weight and a long, disease-free life.

DEFINING DIABETES

Diabetes is an ancient disease written about over 3000 years ago in Egyptian hieroglyphs. The disease called diabetes mellitus comes from diabetes (Greek) for "to pass through" and mellitus (Latin) for "honey sweet." The CDC reports that 29 million Americans have type 2 diabetes while another 89 million have pre-diabetes. Diabetes is the 7th leading cause of death in America the leading cause of adult onset blindness over 650,000 leading cause of kidney failure most diabetics will die from related complications. About half of all diabetics develop neuropathy that can cause numbness, tingling, pain and suffer poor circulation and lack of feeling in the legs and feet which can lead to poorly healing injuries that can in turn end as amputations. Diabetes is the number one cause of death in Mexico and Mexico has been designated by the World Health Organization as the most obese country on earth. China has 92 million type 2 diabetics leading the world. The United Kingdom's Insurance Actuarial tables reflect a shorter life for diabetics.

Diabetes is characterized by chronically elevated levels of sugar in your blood. Insulin is produced in the pancreas (the hormone that keeps your blood sugar in check). With diabetes, you are not producing enough insulin or your body becomes resistant to insulin's effects. Insulin-resistance is called type 2 diabetes. Type 1 is when your immune system kills the insulin producing beta cells.

Your digestive system breaks down carbohydrates you eat into a simple sugar called glucose which is the primary fuel powering all the cells in your body. To get from the bloodstream into your cells, glucose requires insulin. Think of insulin as the key that unlocks the cell's door. Type 1 diabetics do not produce insulin thus they have to inject insulin. A Professor Taylor, formerly of Harvard cell research, has successfully produced beta cells in vitro. Researchers at MIT are hopefully close to perfecting an artificial pancreas. Professor Taylor has a very personal interest since both his adult children have type 1 diabetes.

The Good News: Type 2 diabetes is almost always preventable like other leading killers such as heart disease and high blood pressure. Type 2 diabetes is a consequence of diet; however, if you have diabetes and its complications, there is hope through lifestyle changes. You may be able to achieve a complete remission of type 2 diabetes even if you've been suffering with the disease for decades. Lifestyle changes can start improving your health in a matter of hours.

WHAT CAUSES INSULIN RESISTANCE

Both prediabetes and type 2 diabetes are caused by insulin resistance of the fat toxicity inside of our muscles cells (lipotoxicity) is a major cause of insulin resistance and type 2 diabetes. Insulin resistance can start over a decade before type 2 diabetes is diagnosed. Blood sugar levels slowly start creeping up and then all of a sudden the pancreas conks out and blood sugar skyrockets.

Studies dating back nearly a century note a striking finding. In 1927, researchers divided healthy young medical students into multiple groups to test out the effects of different diets. Some were given a fat-rich diet composed of olive oil, butter, egg yolks, and cream; others were given a carbohydrate-rich diet of sugar, candy, pastry, white bread, baked potatoes, syrup, bananas, rice, and oatmeal. Surprisingly, insulin resistance skyrocketed in the fat-rich diet group. Within a matter of days, their blood sugar levels doubled in response to a sugar challenge, far more than those on the sugar and starch diet.

WHAT UNDERLIES THIS RAPID FAILURE OF INSULIN SECRETION?

At first the pancreas pumps out more and more insulin trying to overcome the fat induced insulin resistance in our muscles. High insulin levels can lead to fat in our liver, called nonalcoholic fatty liver disease, before diagnoses of type 2 diabetes. As fat builds up in our liver, it becomes resistant to insulin too. Normally, the liver is constantly producing blood sugar to keep our brain alive between meals. As soon as we eat the insulin released to deal with the meal normally turns off liver glucose production, which makes sense since we don't need it anymore. Filled with fat the liver becomes insulin resistant like our muscles and so doesn't respond to the meal signal and so it keeps pumping out blood sugar. The pancreas pumps out even more insulin to deal with the high sugars and our liver gets fatter and fatter. That's one of the two vicious cycles of diabetes.

The two twin vicious cycles of diabetes fatty muscles, in the context of too many calories, leads to a fatty liver which leads to an even fattier liver. This is all still before we have diabetes, but then the next vicious cycle starts. Fatty liver can be deadly so the liver starts trying to offload the fat, by dumping it back in the bloodstream in the form of something called VLDL and that starts building up in the cells in the pancreas that produce insulin in the first place. So now we know how diabetes develops.

Fatty muscles lead to a fatty liver, which leads to a fatty pancreas. It's clear that type 2 diabetes is a condition of excess fat inside our organs. The only thing keeping us from diabetes in the first place was the over production of insulin by the pancreas but as fat builds up in the pancreas killing off the beta cells insulin production falls, we're left with the worst of both worlds--insulin resistance combined with a failing pancreas. This is when we get diabetes and may have to start injecting insulin at high levels to overcome the insulin résistance, and these high insulin levels promote cancer. This is one of the reasons obese women get more breast cancer. It all traces back to fat getting into our muscle cells, starting insulin resistance fat from our stomach or fat going into our stomach (the fat you wear or the fat you eat). So now it should make sense why the American Diabetes Association also recommends reduced intake of dietary fats as a strategy for reducing the risk of developing diabetes. (Dr. McDougall's Health & Medical Center, 1970's)

So, fat is jamming up the cell's door preventing insulin from letting glucose enter, more specifically, intramyocelluar lipid the fat inside your muscle cells.

Fat in your bloodstream, either from your own fat stores (you only have so many fat cells when you get fatter and fatter the fat cells become so saturated they spill the fat out into your bloodstream) or the fat you eat. Even among healthy individuals, a high-fat diet can impair the body's ability to handle sugar.

This mechanism by which fat interferes with insulin function has been demonstrated by either infusing fat into people's bloodstreams and watching insulin resistance shoot up or by removing fat from people's blood and seeing insulin resistance drop. They can now even visualize the amount of fat in the muscles using MRI technology. Researchers are now able to track the fat going from the blood into the muscles and watch insulin resistance rise. One hit of fat, and within 160 minutes, the absorption of glucose into your cells become compromised

Professor Roy Taylor of Newcastle University in England, creator of the Newcastle Diet research, indicates individuals have different fat tolerance levels just like people who smoke don't all get lung cancer There is a genetic component and Dr. Neal Barnard, founder of Physicians Committee for Responsible Medicine, explains the genes that effect diabetes are not dictator genes such as the ones that determine your eye color but more like a committee and it's a suggestion which can be trumped by diet and exercise.

Not all fats affect our muscle cells in the same way. Palmitate, the kind of saturated fat found mostly in meat, dairy, and eggs, causes insulin resistance. On the other hand, oleate, the monounsaturated fat found mostly in nuts, olives, and avocados, may actually protect against the detrimental effects of the saturated fat. Saturated fats can wreak all sorts of havoc in muscle cells and may result in the accumulation of more toxic breakdown products (such as ceramide and diacylglycerol) and free radicals and can cause inflammation and even mitochondrial dysfunction—that is, interference with the little power plants (mitochondria) within our cells. This phenomenon is known as lipotoxicity. If we take muscle biopsies from people, saturated fat buildup in the membranes of their muscle cells correlates with insulin resistance. Monounsaturated fats, however, are more likely to be detoxified by the body or safely stored away. (Sweeney, 1927)

CONTRIBUTING RISK FACTORS

Chronic stress causes the release of cortisol. Cortisol provides the body with glucose by tapping into protein stores via gluconeogenesis in the liver. This energy can help an individual fight or flee a stressor. However, elevated cortisol over the long-term consistently produces glucose, leading to increased blood sugar levels.

Theoretically, this mechanism can increase the risk for type 2 diabetes although a causative factor is unknown. Since a principal function of cortisol is to thwart the effect of insulin essentially rendering the cells insulin resistant the body remains in a general insulin resistant state. When cortisol level is chronically elevated overtime, the pancreas struggles to keep up with the high demand for insulin, glucose levels in the blood remain high, the cells cannot get the sugar they need, and the cycle continues. (Marcovecchio & Chiarelli, 2012)

WEIGHT GAIN AND OBESITY

Repeated elevation of cortisol can lead to weight gain. One way is via visceral fat storage. Cortisol can mobilize triglycerides from storage and relocate them to visceral fat cells, deep in the abdomen.

A second way in which cortisol may be involved in weight gain goes back to the blood sugar insulin protein. Consistently high blood glucose levels along with insulin suppression lead to cells that are starved of glucose. But those cells are crying out for energy, and one way to regulate is to send hunger signals to the brain. This can lead to overeating and of course, unused glucose is eventually stored as body fat.

You can have your cortisol levels tested: the adrenal stress index(ASI). The good news is that much can be done to keep cortisol controlled with a Stress Management Anti Inflammation diet. (Marcovecchio, Lucantoni, & Chiarelli, 2011)

Sucralose (Splenda) purpose was to help to mitigate the health risks associated with the national epidemic of obesity. The hope was to provide a healthy sugar substitute. However, that's not how it appears to have turned out with population studies tying consumption of artificial sweeteners, mainly in diet sodas, with increased risk of developing obesity, metabolic syndrome and Type 2 diabetes.

Association is not causation. If you give obese individuals the amount of sucralose found in a can of diet soda, they get a significantly higher blood sugar spike in response to a sugar challenge requiring significantly more insulin; 20% higher insulin levels in the blood, suggesting sucralose causes insulin resistance, this may help to explain the links between artificial sweetener consumption and the development of diabetes, heart disease, and stoke. So, sucralose is not like some inert substance. It affects the blood sugar response. But How?

The Splenda company emphasizes that sucralose is hardly even absorbed in the body and stays in the digestive track to be quickly eliminated from the body. But the fact that it's not absorbed in the small intestine means it makes it down to the large intestine and may affect our gut flora.

They had been studies done on artificial sweeteners with rats but there had never been any human studies until now. They tested saccharin, sucralose, and aspartame, the artificial sweeteners in Sweet & Low, Splenda, and NutraSweet, and found that non-caloric artificial sweeteners induce glucose intolerance by altering the microbes in our gut. The human studies were limited but after a few days on saccharin for example, some people get exaggerated blood sugar responses tied to changes over just one week to the types of bacteria they had in their gut. Acesulfame K, another common artificial sweetencr, was also found subsequently to be associated with changes in gut bacteria.

So all this time artificial sweeteners were meant to stave off chronic diseases but may actually be contributing to the problem due to microbial alterations. Some in the scientific community were surprised that even minor concentrations of a sweetener (they're talking about aspartame) are sufficient to cause substantial changes in gut inhabitants. Others were less surprised. Each molecule of aspartame is after all metabolized into formaldehyde. That may explain why some people who are allergic to formaldehyde have such bad reactions to the stuff. Therefor it's not unexpected that even small amounts might modify bacteria communities. The reports about the safety of aspartame are mixed. All the studies funded by the industry vouched for its' safety, whereas 90% of independently funded studies report that aspartame can cause adverse health effects. And that should tell you something.

Consumers of these food additives which are otherwise perceived as safe, are unaware that these substances may influence their gut bacteria. This may be of particular importance to patients with diseases correlated with modifications of gut bacteria, such as inflammatory bowel diseases like ulcerative colitis and Crohn's disease. These individuals may not realize artificial sweeteners may be affecting their gut. Might the effect be large enough to actually see changes in the incidence of inflammatory bowel disease? Canada was the first country to approve the use of sucralose. What happened to their rates of IBD? Rates did seem to double after the approval of sucralose. What about in the United States? After decades of relatively stable rates of ulcerative colitis and Crohn's disease, rates did appear to start going up. In China, after the approval of sucralose, IBD rates rose 12 fold. Again, these could be total flukes but such correlations were also found on two other continents as well. The good news is, that after stopping artificial sweeteners the original balance of gut bacteria may be restored within weeks. Now of course the negative consequences of artificial sweeteners should not be interpreted to suggest we should all go back to sugar and high fructose corn syrup. For optimal health it is recommended that we all try to cut down on both. (Bokulich & Blaser, 2014)

EGGS AND DIABETES

We know the consumption of eggs is associated with the development of some other chronic diseases. What about diabetes? Researchers found a stepwise increase in risk the more and more eggs people ate. Eating just a single egg a week appeared to increase the odds of diabetes by 76%. Two eggs a week appeared to double the odds, and just a single egg a day tripled the odds. Three times greater risk of type 2 diabetes, one of the leading causes of death and amputation, blindness and kidney failure. This is not the first time a link between eggs and diabetes has been reported. In 2009, Harvard researchers found that a single egg a day or more was associated with an increased risk of type 2 diabetes in men and women, and that finding has also been confirmed in other populations: Asia in 2011 and Europe in 2012. And the high consumption of eggs associated with diabetes risk was less than one a day. Through it appears you have to start early once you get into your 70s avoiding eggs may not help. Once we have diabetes, eggs may hasten our death. Eating one egg a day appears to shorten anyone's lifespan, but may double the all-cause mortality for those with diabetes. Not good news for the egg industry. From a transcript of a closed meeting Dr. Michael Greger got through the Freedom of information act "Given the rate at which obesity and incidence of type 2 diabetes" is growing in the United States "any association between dietary cholesterol and type 2 diabetes" "could be a 'showstopper' that could overshadow" "the positive attributes (of) eggs." Another Freedom of Information request showed that The United States Department of Agriculture would not allow egg producers (using government funds set aside for egg promotion) to advertise that eggs were safe or even healthy but they could say they were fresh. (Radzevičienė & Ostrauskas, 2012)

WHY IS MEAT A RISK FACTOR FOR DIABETES?

It has been acknowledged that being overweight and obesity are important risk factor for type 2 diabetes mellitus. A 2013 meta-analysis of all the cohorts looking at meat and diabetes found significantly higher risk associated with total meat consumption, and especially processed meat, particularly poultry. But Why?

There's a whole list of potential culprits in meat. Maybe it's the saturated fat and animal fat. Maybe it's the trans fats that are naturally found in meat. Maybe it's the cholesterol or the animal protein. The heme iron in meat can lead to free radicals, and this iron-induced oxidative stress iron may lead to chronic inflammation, type 2 diabetes. Advanced glycation end products are another problem. They promote oxidative stress and inflammation, and food analyses show that the highest levels of these so-called glycotoxins are found in meat, particularly roasted, fried, or broiled meat, though any foods from animal sources can be potent sources of these pro-oxidant chemicals. In this study they fed diabetics foods packed with glycotoxins, like chicken, fish, and eggs, and their inflammatory markers shot up: tumor necrosis factor, C-reactive protein, vascular adhesion molecules. Thus, in diabetes, dietary AGEs promote inflammatory mediators, leading to tissue injury.The good news though is that restriction of these kinds of foods may suppress these inflammatory effects.

Appropriate measures to limit AGE intake, such as eliminating these foods or sticking to just steaming and boiling meat, may greatly reduce the already heavy burden of these toxins in the diabetic patient. These glycotoxins may be the missing link between the increased consumption of animal fat and meats and the development of type 2 diabetes in the first place.

Since the 2013 meta-analysis was published, this study came out, in which about 17000 people were followed for about a dozen years. They found an 8% increased risk for every 50 grams of daily meat consumption. So that's just like a quarter of a chicken breast worth of meat for the entire day may significantly increase risk of diabetes. Yes, it could be the glycotoxins in meat, or the saturated fat, or the trans-fat in meat, or the heme iron, which could actually promote the formation of carcinogens called nitrosamines though they could also just be produced in the cooking process itself, but this is new.

There appears to be a clear excess of diabetes in those that handle meat for a living. Maybe there's some kind of diabetes causing zoonotic infectious agent like viruses present in fresh cuts of meat, including poultry. Over-stimulation of the aging enzyme TOR pathway by excess food consumption may be a crucial factor underlying the diabetes epidemic, but not just any food. Animal proteins may not only stimulate the cancer-promoting growth hormone IGF-1, but provide high amounts of leucine, which stimulates TOR activation, and appears to burn out the insulin producing beta cells in the pancreas and contribute to type 2 diabetes. So it's not just the high fat and added sugars. Critical attention has to be paid to the daily intake of animal proteins.

In general, lower leucine levels are only really reached by the restriction of animal proteins. We now have experimental evidence that exposure to industrial toxins alone induces weight gain and therefore may be an underappreciated cause of obesity and diabetes. Consider what's happening to our infants. Obesity in a six-month old is not related to diet or lack of exercise. They're now exposed to hundreds of chemicals from their moms, straight through the umbilical cord, some of which may be obesogenic - obesity generated. Given the millions of pounds of chemicals and heavy metals released every year into the environment, it should make us all stop and think about how we live and the choices we make every day in the food we eat. This 2014 review of the evidence on pollutants and diabetes noted, yes we can be exposed through some toxic spill, but most of human exposure nowadays is from the ingestion of contaminated food as a results of bioaccumulation up the food chain. And the main source, around 95%, of persistent pollutant intake is through dietary intake of animal fat. (Hyman, 2010)

DIABETES AND DIOXINS

Finding higher diabetes rates among those heavily exposed to toxic pollutants-chemical plant explosions, living next to a toxic waste dump, or eating fish out of the Great Lakes-that's one thing, but would the same link be found in just a random sample of the general population? Yes, a strong dose-dependent relationship between the levels of these pollutants circulating in people's blood and diabetes. Those with the highest levels of pollutants in their blood stream had 38 times the odds of diabetes. Interestingly, there was no association between obesity and diabetes among subjects with non- levels of pollutants. In other words, obesity was a risk factor for diabetes only if people had blood concentrations of these pollutants above a certain level. We all know obesity predisposes us to diabetes, but according to this study, only if our bodies are polluted, only perhaps if the fat we're carrying is carrying chemicals.

This finding kind of implies that virtually all the risk of diabetes conferred by obesity is attributable to these pollutants, and that obesity might only be a vehicle for such chemicals. Could we be carrying around our own little toxic waste dump on our hips? This possibility is shocking. Now it's entirely possible that the six pollutants they looked at are not themselves causally related to diabetes. Maybe they're just surrogates of exposure to a mixture of chemicals. After all, 90% of these pollutants come from animal foods in the general population. Except for individuals living or working around industrial sites where these chemicals were used or dumped the most common source of exposure to PCBs is from diet, with foods of animal origin, especially seafood, so this strong relationship they found between certain pollutants and diabetes may just be pointing to other contaminants in animal products. (Hyman, 2010)

STATIN DRUGS

February 28, 2012 the FDA announced newly mandated safety labeling for cholesterol lowering statin drugs, such as Lipitor, Mevacor, Crestor, Zocor, and Vytorins. The FDA issued new side effect warnings regarding the increased risk of brain-related side effects such as memory loss and confusion, and an increase in blood sugar levels and risk of new onset diabetes associated with taking this class of drugs

One prominent cardiologist described the Faustian bargain to the Wall Street Journal. Apparently one to two out of 100 patients at risk for heart attack will avoid one by taking statins but research now suggests for every 200 people taking a statin, one will develop diabetes. The third side effect, newly addressed by the FDA the risk of muscle injury. They've known that about 1-5% of patients suffer enough muscle damage to cause pain and overt weakness, but only about one in 6 or 7 million actually suffers enough muscle damage to kill them. It's called fatal rhabdomyolysis, where your muscles break down so rapidly your urine starts looking like brown Kool-Aid. You literally start peeing your muscles down the toilet, then your kidneys fail and you die. But those are lottery odds there's a 1 in 2 chance we'll die of heart disease, so no surprise Lipitor is the #1 prescribed drug on the planet Earth.

Then this study was published: Normally if you have muscle pain on a statin, you go to a doctor and they take blood to see if you have elevated levels of muscle breakdown products in your bloodstream. And if you don't, they basically say, oh, it's all in your head, go home and keep taking your medicine. But these researchers instead took these people and got muscle biopsies and proved that even though their blood levels were normal they were indeed suffering muscle damage. The damage just wasn't leaking into their blood stream. Well, if that's the case, if you can't pick it up with the test, maybe everyone taking statins is suffering muscle damage, whether they're experiencing pain or not. And that's exactly what they found. Clear evidence of skeletal muscle damage in statin-treated patients -all statin-treated patients. The degree of overall damage was slight. Most people don't even feel any pain with statins, so what's the big deal? This is the big deal. A study on statins therapy muscle function and falls risk. Hundreds of older men and women were followed for a few years, and those who were on statins suffered greater declines in muscle strength and muscle quality, and greater increases in falls risk. So we don't want to be taking this drug unless we really need it. The problem is because heart disease remains our #1 killer most everyone does need to take a statin drug like Lipitor every day for the rest of their lives, except for one group. This is from the Editor in Chief of the American Journal of Cardiology. Only pure vegetarians do not need statins most of the rest of us do so it's our choice. (The U.S. Food and Drug Administration (FDA), 2012)

I stopped taking statins the day I read the FDA warning: I was flushing my muscle down the toilet, thought I had cancer and was attempting to increase my life insurance when I read the FDA warning. The only warning on my Lipitor was don't consume grapefruits, dilutes the statins effectiveness.

DRUGS, DIET, AND EXERCISE TO CONTROL DIABETES

The higher the blood sugar level the higher the risk for more heart attacks, strokes, shorter life span and higher risk of complications like blindness and kidney failure.

A study was designed where 10,000 diabetics were randomized into an intensive blood sugar lowering intervention, where they put people on up to 5 different classes of drugs with or without insulin to drive blood sugar down into the normal range. They are not treating the underlying cause, not treating the actual disease, but lowering the effects of the disease by any means necessary. The hope was to prevent some of the devastating complications.

How did it work? The intensive blood sugar lowering with drugs increased mortality. The harm associated with increased risk of death outweighed any potential benefits and they stopped the study prematurely for safety reasons. They were successful in bringing people's blood sugar down. Maybe the increase in mortality with an intensive glucose lowering strategy could have been related to the adverse effects of the drugs. Even just injected insulin itself may promote cancer, obesity, atherosclerosis, worsen diabetic retinopathy, and accelerate aging. Insulin therapy may promote inflammation in the lining of our arteries, which may help explain the results of this trial and other trials like it that showed the same thing--no reductions in so-called macrovascular complications, heart attack, and strokes, with intensive blood sugar lowering. These trials relied exclusively on drugs with no diet or lifestyle changes.

A 2013 paper in the New England Journal of Medicine, "Cardiovascular Effects of Intensive Lifestyle Intervention in Type 2 Diabetes" states that focusing on weight loss did not decrease the rate of cardiovascular events in overweight or obese adults with type 2 diabetes it did not lower their risk of death but it did not increase the risk of death. In fact, the trial was stopped after about 10 years on the basis of futility since they lost weight but they weren't dying any less.

Other trials had similar results. Why was this not helping people live longer? Because they didn't put them on a healthier diet. They just put them on a smaller diet, a calorie restricted diet, meaning the same lousy diet just smaller portions. If we eat less and exercise more we can lose weight, get more physically fit, slimmer and have better blood sugar control, but if our diets continue to be so non-heart-healthy that our bad LDL cholesterol doesn't improve then we're not going to be unclogging our arteries.

Whereas individuals following healthier diets may experience improved reductions of blood sugar, body weight and cardiovascular risk, which is the point of a lifestyle intervention not so we can fit in smaller caskets.

HOW TO PREVENT PRE-DIABETES
FROM BECOMING DIABETES

The Centers for Disease Control and Prevention predicts by 2050 one out of every three of us may have diabetes. The consequences of diabetes are #1 cause of adult-onset blindness in adults 20-74 years, the #1 cause of kidney failure, the #1 cause of surgical amputations. What can we do to prevent it?

The onset of type 2 diabetes is gradual, with most individuals progressing through a state of prediabetes, a condition now striking approximately 1 in 3 Americans, but only about 1 in 10 even knows it. Since current methods of treating diabetes remain inadequate, prevention is preferable, but what works better? Lifestyle changes or drugs. We didn't know until this landmark study was published in New England Journal of Medicine.

Thousands were randomized to get a good double dose of the leading anti-diabetes drug or diet and exercise. The drug metformin is probably the safest diabetes drug there is. It does cause diarrhea in about half of those who take it, makes 1 in 4 nauseous, about 1 in 10 suffer from asthenia, meaning lack of strength, causing physical weakness and fatigue, but the risk of being killed by the drug is only about 1 in 66,000 every year. And the drug worked compared to placebo, in terms of the percentage of people developing diabetes in the 4-year study period fewer people in the drug group developed diabetes. But diet and exercise alone worked better. The lifestyle intervention reduced diabetes incidence by 58%, compared to only 31% with the drug.

The lifestyle intervention was significantly more effective than the drug, and had fewer side-effects. More than three quarters of those on the drug reported gastrointestinal symptoms, though there was more muscle soreness reported in the lifestyle group, on account they were actually exercising. Other studies subsequently found the same result: non-drug approaches superior to drug-based approaches for diabetes prevention. And the 50% or so drop in risk was not for people that actually improved their diet and lifestyle, but just for those instructed to improve their diet and lifestyle, whether or not they actually did it.

Pay Attention: this is one of the most famous diabetes prevention studies. 500 people with pre-diabetes randomized into a lifestyle intervention or control group, and during the trial, the risk of diabetes was reduced by that same 50-60%, but only a fraction of the patients met the modest goals. Even in the lifestyle intervention group, only about a quarter were able to eat enough fiber, meaning whole plant foods and cut down on enough saturated fat, which in this country is mostly dairy, dessert, chicken, and pork. But they did better than the control group and fewer of them developed diabetes because of it.

But what if you looked just at the folks that actually made the lifestyle changes, met at least 4 out of 5 of those wimpy goals? They had ZERO diabetes. None of them got diabetes. A 100% drop in risk. Bottom line: type 2 diabetes can be prevented by changes in lifestyle even in high-risk pre-diabetic subjects. The fact, then, that type 2 diabetes, a largely preventable disorder, has reached such epidemic proportion is a public health humiliation. (Greger, 2014)

GOALS TO PREVENT PRE-DIABETES FROM BECOMING DIABETIC

- Weight Reduction > 7%

- Fat intake > 30% of energy intake

- Saturated Fat intake > 10% of energy intake

- Fiber intake >15 grams / 1000 Kcal and Exercise >4.hours a week

Turmeric Curcumin for Prediabetes is an extraordinary study was published in the Journal of the American Diabetes Association. Curcumin extract for prevention of type 2 diabetes. A randomized, double-blinded placebo-controlled trial of folks diagnosed with prediabetes.

Half got supplements of curcumin, the yellow pigment in the spice turmeric and curry powder, and the other half got identical looking placebos, and they just followed them out for nine months to see who ended up with diabetes. After nine months of treatment, 16% of subjects in the placebo group went on to get full-blown diabetes. How many in the curcumin group? None! The curcumin group saw a significant improvement in fasting blood sugars, glucose tolerance, hemoglobin A1C, insulin sensitivity, pancreatic insulin-producing beta cell function (measured two different ways), and insulin sensitivity. What if you already have diabetes? Same beneficial effects, at a fraction of the dose. The prediabetes study used the equivalent, like a quarter cup of turmeric a day. Whereas this group used only about a teaspoon's worth, which is doable through diet rather than supplements. What's interesting is the purported mechanism. Fat in the bloodstream plays an important role in the development of insulin resistance and ultimately, type 2 diabetes. Fat builds up inside your muscle cells and gums up the works, all the inflammation, interfering with insulin signaling. This is the first study that shows that these turmeric spice compounds may have an anti-diabetic effect by decreasing fats in the blood. So if you are pre-diabetic, it might be a good idea to add turmeric to your diet. But it's important to recognize that prediabetes is a disease in itself, increasing the risk of death, cancer, heart disease, and vision loss. So it's not enough to just prevent progression to full-blown diabetes, prediabetes may be cured completely, with a healthy plant-based diet.

LIFESTYLE MEDICINE IS THE STANDARD OF CARE FOR PREDIABETES

Lifestyle modifications is now considered the cornerstone of diabetes prevention. Diet-wise that means individuals with prediabetes or diabetes, diabetes should aim to reduce their intake of excess calories, saturated fat, and trans fat. Too many of us consume a diet with too many of these solid fats as well as added sugars. Thankfully the latest dietary guidelines aim to shift consumption towards more plant-based foods. Lifestyle modification is now the foundation of the American Association of Clinical Endocrinology guidelines, the European Diabetes Association guidelines, as well as the official standards of care for the American Diabetes Association.

Dietary strategies include reduced intake of fat, and increased intake of fiber, meaning unrefined plant foods including whole grains. We've known eating lots of whole grains is associated with a reduced risk of developing type 2 diabetes. A recent study took it further, demonstrating that whole grain consumption may also protect against prediabetes in the first place.

To help prevent diabetics from dying, recommendations should focus on the reduction of saturated fat, cholesterol, and trans fat intake, which is basically code for meat and dairy, eggs, and junk food, and increases in omega 3's, soluble fiber, and phytoserols, all of which can be found packaged in flax seeds, for example, an efficient but still uncommon intervention for prediabetes. They found that about 2 tablespoons of ground flax a day decrease insulin resistance, which is the hallmark of the disease.

CURING DIABETIC NEUROPATHY

Neuropathy, or damage to the nerves, is a debilitating disorder. Diabetes is by far the common cause, and up to 50% of patients will eventually develop neuropathy during the course of their disease. It can be very painful and the pain is frequently resistant to conventional treatments. In fact, there is currently no effective treatment for diabetic neuropathy.

But in the early 80's researchers in Southern California published a remarkable study on the regression of diabetic neuropathy with a plant-based diet. This study took twenty-one diabetics suffering with moderate or worse symptomatic painful neuropathy for up to ten years and placed them on a whole-foods, plant-based diet along with a half-hour walk every day.

Years and years of suffering and then, complete relief of the pain for 17 out of the 21 patients within days. Numbness noticeably improved too. And the side-effects were all good. They lost ten pounds, blood sugars got better, insulin needs dropped in half, and five of the patients not only apparently had their painful neuropathy cured, so was their diabetes--normal blood sugars and off of all medications. And their triglycerides and cholesterol improved too. High blood pressure got better too. In fact, about half the hypertensives experienced an 80% drop overall in the need for high blood pressure medications with three weeks. This was a live-in program where patients' meals were provided. What happened after they were sent home? The 17 folks were followed for years, and in all except one, the relief from the painful neuropathy continued or improved even further. How'd they get that kind of compliance? Pain and ill health are strong motivating factors.

One of the most painful and frustrating conditions to treat in all of medicine and 75% cured in a couple days with a natural nontoxic-in fact beneficial-treatment, a diet composed of whole, plant foods. How could nerve damage be reversed so suddenly? It wasn't the improvement in blood sugar control since it took about ten days for the diet to control the diabetes, whereas the pain was gone in as few as four. Several mechanisms by which the total vegetarian diet works to alleviate the problem of diabetic neuropathy as well as the diabetic condition itself. One interesting speculation was that it could be the trans fats naturally found in meat and dairy and refined vegetable oils that could be causing an inflammatory response. They found a significant percentage of the fat found under the skin of those who ate meat or dairy consisted of trans fats, where those on a strictly whole food plant-based diet had none.

They stuck needles in the buttocks of people eating different diets, and nine months or more on a strict plant-based diet appeared to remove the trans fats from their bodies ... at least their butts. But their pain didn't take nine months to get better--it got better in days. More likely it was due to an improvement in blood flow. Nerve biopsies in diabetics with severe progressive neuropathy have shown small vessel disease within the nerve. There are blood vessels within our nerves that can get clogged up. The oxygen levels in the nerves of diabetics were found to be lower than even that of de-oxygenated blood. This lack of oxygen within the nerve may arise from blockages within the blood vessels depriving the nerve oxygen, presumably leading them to cry out in pain. Within days, though, improvements in blood rheology, the ease of blood flow on a plant-based diet may play a prominent role in the reversal of diabetic neuropathy. Plant based diets may lower the levels of IGF-1 inside the eyeballs of diabetics and decrease the risk of retinopathy-diabetic vision loss-as well. But the most efficient way to avoid diabetic complications is to eliminate the diabetes, and this is often feasible for those type 2 patients who make an abiding commitment to daily exercise and a healthy enough diet. Since the initial report of neuropathy reversal, the results have been replicated, significant improvements in numbness and burning. Why don't doctors learn about this in medical school? The neglect of this important work by the broader medical community is nothing short of unconscionable.

The National Academy of Sciences, one of the most prestigious institution in the world, "advisors to the nation," responding to the question how much trans fat is safe, answered "Zero." The FDA has banned the use of trans fat and it will be phased out over the next couple of years except in meat where it occurs naturally.

REVERSING AND CURING DIABETES

Doctors noticed that reducing the size of the stomach cured type 2 diabetes (Bariatric Gastric By-pass Surgery). These surgical results led to the Newcastle Diabetes Reversal research. Prof Taylor attempted to mimic the effects of gastric bypass surgery without actually doing any surgery. He put 11 diabetics on a very low calorie diet, 600 Kcal per day, for 8 weeks. The result was that glucose levels and insulin response became non- diabetic in all the patients. Their insulin response became supernormal after 8 weeks. Even better than those having the surgery.

What Happened? Remember, Type 2 diabetes can be understood as a potentially reversible metabolic state precipitated by the single cause of chronic excess intra-organ fat: too much fat in the liver, pancreas, and muscles. Within 7 days of instituting a substantial negative calorie balance by either dietary intervention or bariatric surgery, fasting plasma glucose levels can normalize. This rapid change relates to a substantial fall in liver fat content and return of normal hepatic insulin sensitivity. Over 8 weeks, first phase and maximal rate of insulin secretion steadily return too normal, and this change is in step with steadily decreasing pancreatic fat content.

So if the cause of diabetes goes away then the diabetes goes away. The insulin producing beta cells of the pancreas had woken up. This has never been demonstrated before. Clearly, the B-cells are not permanently damaged in Type 2 diabetes, but are merely metabolically inhibited.   They report reversal of diabetes in patients up to 28 years after diagnoses. So diabetics motivated enough to starve themselves can regain normal health. This information should be available to all people with diabetes. Even though with present methods of changing eating habits, it is unlikely that weight loss can be achieved in those not strongly motivated to escape from diabetes.

They should know that if it is not reversed, the consequences for future health and cost are dire, although these serious adverse effects must be balanced against the difficulties and privations associated with a substantial and sustained change in eating patterns. What about Bariatric surgery? Major surgery has major risk such as deep vein thrombosis, pulmonary embolism and pneumonia. Specific morbidities associated with the gastric band include vomiting, band slippage and erosion, esophageal dilatation and development of a gastric pouch. There may also be problems with the band such as secretion, leaks and abdominal port disconnection requiring band change.   With diversionary operations, there is risk of bleeding, anastomotic leakage, herniation, gastric pouch dilatation, severe nutritional deficiencies, and dumping syndrome. Major surgery, you get major risk.

WHAT ABOUT TREATING DIABETES WITH HEALTHIER FOOD?

Successful treatment of diabetes with a plant-based diet goes back to the 1930's--not eating less food but healthier food--90 percent or more plant-based diet of all-you-can-eat greens, lots of other vegetables and beans, whole grains, fruits at every meal, nuts, and seeds; to restrict their animal product consumption; and to eliminate refined grains, junk food, and oil.

Researchers took a group of diabetics and put them on plant-based diet and measured their hemoglobin A1c levels considered the best measure of how poorly blood sugars have been controlled over time.

At the onset of the study, the diabetics had A1c levels averaging 8.2. An A1c level under 5.7 is considered normal, between 5.7 and 6.4 is considered prediabetics, and above 6.5 is considered diabetic. However, the American Diabetes Association's target is just to get most diabetics down below 7.0 (recall that intensive blood-sugar-lowering trials using drugs, which tried to push A1c levels under 6.0, unfortunately ended up increasing the mortality rate).

After about seven months of eating a diet centered on whole plant foods, the subjects' A1c levels dropped to a nondiabetic 5.8—and this was after they were able to stop taking most of their medications. Now we know diabetes can be reversed on an extremely healthy diet, but is that because it was also low in calories? The study subjects lost about as much weight on the vegetable-packed plant-based diet as people who went on semi starvation diets. But even if this type of diabetes reversal was just about calorie restriction, which one would be healthier and sustainable?

Surprisingly, even participants who temporarily didn't lose weight on the plant based diet, or who actually gained weight, still appeared to improve their diabetes. In other words, the beneficial effects of plant-based diets may extend beyond weight loss. However, the study described just a handful of people, had no control group, and included only those who could stick to the eating plan. To prove plant-based diets could actually improve diabetes independent of weight loss, researchers would need to design a study in which they switched people to a healthy diet but forced them to eat so much that they didn't lose any weight.

Just such a study was published more than thirty-five years ago. Type 2 diabetics were placed on a plant-based diet and weighed every day. If they started losing any weight, they were made to eat more food—so much that some of the participants actually had trouble eating it all!

The Results: Even with no weight loss, subjects on the plant-based diet saw their insulin requirements cut by about 60%, meaning the amount of insulin these diabetics had to inject dropped by more than half. Furthermore, half of the diabetics were able to get off insulin altogether, despite no change in body weight—just by eating a healthier diet.

This wasn't over the course of months or years, either. This was after eating a plant-based diet for an average of only sixteen days. Some of the subjects had been diabetic for two decades and had been injecting twenty units of insulin a day. Yet within two weeks of eating a plant-based diet, they were off insulin altogether. One patient was on thirty-two units of insulin per day at the onset of the study. After eighteen days, his blood sugar levels plummeted so low that insulin injections were no longer necessary. Even at approximately the same body weight, he had lower blood sugars on a plant-based diet using no insulin than when he had been on a regular diet using thirty-two units of insulin daily. That's the power of plants. And as a bonus, their cholesterol dropped like a rock, in 16 days.

HOW CAN PLANTS PROTECT AGAINST DIABETES AND MEAT CONSUMPTION BE A RISK FACTOR FOR DIABETES?

There appears to be a stepwise reduction in diabetes rate as meat consumption drops. Rather than something they're avoiding in meat, it may be something people are getting from plants. Free radicals may be the important trigger for insulin resistance, so antioxidants in plant foods may help. Put people on a plant-based diet and their antioxidant enzymes shoot up, so not only do plants provide antioxidants but boost our own endogenous antioxidant defenses, where on a conventional diabetic diet they get worse. There are phytonutrients in plant foods that may help lower chronic disease prevalence by acting as antioxidants, anti-cancer agents, and lowering cholesterol and blood sugar. Some we're now theorizing, may even be lipotropes, meaning they have the capacity to hasten the removal of fat from our organs like the liver, thereby counteracting the inflammatory cascade believed to be directly initiated by saturated fat containing foods. Fat in the bloodstream, due to the fat we wear or the fat we eat not only causes insulin resistance, but produces a low-grade inflammation that can contribute to heart disease and non-alcoholic fatty liver disease. Fiber may also decrease insulin resistance. One of the ways it may do that is by helping to rid the body of excess estrogen. There is strong evidence for a direct role of estrogens in the cause of diabetes, and it's demonstrated that certain gut bacteria can produce estrogens in our colon. High-fat low-fiber diets appear to stimulate the metabolic activity of these estrogen-producing intestinal bacteria. This is a problem for men too. Obesity is associated with low testosterone levels, marked elevations of estrogens, produced not only by fat cells but some of the bacteria in our gut. Our intestinal bacteria may produce these so called diabetogens, diabetes-causing compounds, from the fats that we eat. By eating lots of fiber though, we can flush this excess estrogen out of our bodies. Vegetarian women, for example excrete two to three times more estrogens in their feces than omnivorous women, which may be why the omnivorous women had 50% higher estrogen blood levels. These differences in estrogen metabolism may help explain the lower incidence of diabetes in those eating more plant-based diets, as well as the lower incidence of breast cancer in vegetarian woman, who get rid of twice as much estrogen because they get rid of twice as much daily waste in general. Either way, meat consumption is consistently associated with diabetes risk. Dietary habits are readily modifiable, individuals and clinicians will consider dietary changes only if they are aware of the potential benefits of doing so. The identification of meat consumption as a risk factor for diabetes provides helpful guidance that can set the stage for beneficial behavioral changes. Meat consumption is something doctors can readily identify. Once identified, at-risk individuals can then be encouraged to familiarize themselves with meatless options. Meat protein makes your insulin go up as much as pure sugar.

Just like moderate changes in diet usually result in only modest reductions in cholesterol, asking people with diabetes to make moderate changes often achieves equally moderate results, which is one possible reason why most end up on drugs, injections, or both. It's your choice.

Diet	BMI (body mass index) over 30 is considered obese	Diabetes Risk
SAD - Standard American Diet	average BMI 28.8	
Flexitarian - plant-based with occasional inclusion of meat	BMI 27.3	28% lower
Vegetarian	BMI 25.7	61% lower
Vegan	BMI 23.6	78% lower

40lbs difference between vegan and those eating SAD on average

NEWCASTLE LOW CALORIE DIET PROGRAM (700 CALORIES PER DAY)

- Meal replacement with Optifast (3 sachets each day)-this provides a total of 600 calories and the necessary daily vitamins and mineral requirements

- Eat up to 3 portions of non-starch vegetables each day (total of 250g each day) (for fiber content) – this will provide another 200 calories

- Drink – liters of water or calorie-free beverages each day

- During the 8 weeks of the diet;

- No poultry or fish or meat

- No bread or pasta

- No dairy products (even full skimmed milk!)

- No root vegetables like potato, sweet potato, turnip

- No pulses

- No fruits

- No alcohol

- During the first few days of the diet, you may experience some symptoms like

- Headache

- Dizziness

- Tiredness

- Hunger

- Cold

These are expected as your body adjust to using your fat store as energy source.

The symptoms will improve after 2-4 days. It is important to keep up your fluid intake and remember to wrap up warmly! The problem is this is a diet and temporary most people who lose weight on fad diets gain it back as did several diabetics in the study along with their diabetes. You have to change your lifestyle for long term health and that means a more wholefood plant based diet and exercise.

The creator of cureddiabetes.com tried the Newcastle Diet lost weight but did not cure his diabetes. He developed his own program of low carbs and exercise and reversed his diabetes, His A1c was over 11 now it's below 5. Gordon was not obese. Some go on a 5-2 diet eating normal 5 days a week and doing the Newcastle Diet on two nonconsecutive days. Gordon's low carb diet and exercise consist of eating less than 50 grams of carb a day and walking down your blood sugar after a meal to 90 and building muscle with resistance training. Gordon is a Cambridge mathematics scholar and scientist. He helps type 2 diabetics who are not on insulin. His definition of cured is being able to pass a glucose tolerance test on a hundred grams of carbs and one hour of exercise a day which is the minimum one should do anyway.

Researchers found that cardiovascular disease incidence more than doubled in the low-carb, high-protein followers. American Kidney Fund warns about impact of high-protein diets on kidney health and Dr. Paul W. Crawford, M.D. AKF Chair of Medical Affairs, worries that strain put on the kidneys could result in irreversible "scarring in the Kidneys." He also warned high protein diets for bodybuilders could be predisposing themselves to chronic kidney disease because hyper filtration (the strain on the kidneys) can produce scarring in the kidneys, reducing kidney function."

Dr. Crawford concluded, "Chronic kidney disease is not to be taken lightly, and there is no cure for kidney failure. The only treatments are kidney dialysis and kidney transplantation. This research shows that even in healthy athletes, kidney function was impacted and that ought to send a message to anyone who is on a high-protein weight loss diet."

Gordon encourages vegetable consumption and a low carb diet, not meat based, can be healthy. His site is full of useful information and success stories.

With the whole food plant based diet you lose weight relatively quickly, comparable to gastric bypass surgery or the New Castle starvation diet. I was diagnosed with diabetes in November of 2014 and discovered statins had given me rhabdomyolysis, where your muscles breakdown so rapidly your urine starts looking like brown Kool-Aid, so I stopped taking them.

You are feeling tired due to having high sugar and exercise will reduce that sugar level. Here is how you fix your muscles. First, you walk for 30 minutes to floor your sugar. Then you do high Intensity Exercise. Not on your legs! You will not be able to run the next day. Check with a doctor before doing high Intensity exercise!

December 1, 2014 I started the diet my A1C was 7.6. Mild diabetes my diabetic neuropathy cleared up by December 10. Then I knew everything I had read was true. January 15, 2015 A1c 5.7and weight loss of a little over 20 pounds. Dr. Neal Barnard says, "Preventing and reversing diabetes is not all about weight loss. The nutritional features of this diet have profound effects on improving pancreatic function and lowering insulin resistance over and above what could be accomplished with weight loss alone." The amazing thing is you continue to lose weight until you get to your healthy weight and you remain at that healthy weight as long as you eat a predominant plant based diet. I didn't count calories. I didn't measure servings. Fruit was limited to 4 or 5 servings but compared to what-- how many servings of fruit did I have before.

This is the only approach that lowers cholesterol, lowers triglycerides, and lowers blood pressure as it drops weight and blood glucose. Pritikin had alumnus from the Pritikin longevity center diabetic for 20 years taking 80 unites of insulin a day off all insulin in 6 weeks with better blood sugar. If you are on medication for diabetes, you need to be under a physician's supervision for this dietary intervention and closely follow your blood glucose and blood pressure.

EXERCISE

I walked after every meal until my blood sugar was down to 90. I would walk 30 minutes at 4 mph, check my blood sugar, and, if necessary. walk another 30 minutes and do resistance training and High Intensity Exercise every other day. When I stopped the statins, the pain stopped. Since May 2015 my A1c is 5.1. I jog 45 minutes in the morning at 6mph and resistance train most afternoons. I recommend everyone have a home treadmill and join a health club.

- Gordon Richie creator of the cureddiabetes.com

- Diabetes progresses when your A1C is above 6.0%

- Diabetes regresses when your A1C is below 5.5%

There are so many ways in which diabetes fights against you when you try and cure it.

- It gives you neuropathy in the feet which makes it hard and painful to walk

- It raises your blood sugar so that exercise does not improve your muscle mass but merely burns off the excess sugar

- It makes you feel tired. You think that you do not have the energy to exercise but you do. You have loads of sugar to burn.

The trick is to realize that your body is sick. It is sending you the wrong signals. If you feel tired as a diabetic, then exercise and you will feel less tired! It is true.

Vol.2, No.3, 364-371 (2012)
http://dx.doi.org/10.4236/ojpm.2012.23053

Glycemic and cardiovascular parameters improved in type 2 diabetes with the high nutrient density (HND) diet

D. M. Dunaief[1], J. Fuhrman[2*], J. L. Dunaief[3], G. Ying[4]

[1]Private Practice, Medical Compass MD, East Setauket, USA
[2]Private Practice, Flemington, USA; *Corresponding Author: mdoffice@drfuhrman.com
[3]F.M. Kirby Center for Molecular Ophthalmology, University of Pennsylvania, Philadelphia, PA, USA
[4]Center for Preventive Ophthalmology and Biostatistics, Perelman School of Medicine, University of Pennsylvania, Philadelphia, USA

Received 6 April 2012; revised 26 May 2012; accepted 8 June 2012

ABSTRACT

Objective: The purpose of this study was to provide an initial assessment of the effectiveness of the high nutrient density (HND) diet on glycemic control and cardiovascular risk factors in participants with type 2 diabetes. Design: This was a retrospective case series study. Participants were 13 adult type 2 diabetic U.S. women and men between the ages of 30 - 80 years old. Glycosylated hemoglobin (HbA1C), lipid profile, blood pressure, BMI, and medication requirements before and after commencement of the HND diet were compared. Results: After a median length on the HND diet of 7 months, the mean HbA1C dropped from 8.2% to 5.8% (p = 0.002), with sixty-two percent of participants reaching normoglycemic levels (HbA1C < 6.0%). There was a substantial reduction in mean blood pressure for hypertensive participants (n=10) from a pre-intervention level of 148/87 mmHg to 121/74 mmHg (p = 0.0004 for systolic blood pressure, p = 0.01 for diastolic blood pressure). Triglycerides significantly decreased from a mean of 171 mg/dl to a mean of 103 mg/dl (p = 0.02). The mean HDL increased significantly from 48.3 mg/dl to 54.6 mg/dl (p = 0.03). The mean number of medications dropped from 4 to 1 (p = 0.0006). Conclusions: The HND diet was very effective in controlling glycemic levels and cardiovascular risk factors in 13 participants with type 2 diabetes. Therefore, there is a well-justified need for further study with the HND diet.

Keywords: Type 2 Diabetes Mellitus; Lipids; Hypertension; Nutrition; Cardiovascular Disease; Lifestyle Medicine; HbA1C; BMI

1. INTRODUCTION

Lowering complication risk and achieving better metabolic control are the central goals of medical care for type 2 diabetes, but outcomes are inconsistent. In the 2009 consensus statement of the American Diabetes Association (ADA) and the European Association for the Study of Diabetes, the organizations recommend starting a nascent type 2 diabetes patient on lifestyle changes plus metformin. According to the authors, for most individuals, lifestyle interventions fail to achieve or maintain the metabolic goals [1]. Only about 37% of type 2 diabetes patients in 1999-2000 Third National Health and Nutrition Examination Survey have achieved the ADA's recommended goal of a HbA1C < 7.0% [2].

Diets low in animal protein and saturated fat and high in complex carbohydrates, fiber and micronutrients improve glucose tolerance, postprandial glucose and overall glycemic control, as well as decrease insulin resistance [3-7]. The high nutrient density (HND) diet emphasizes micronutrients (phytochemicals and antioxidants) from greens, fruits, nuts/seeds and beans/legumes, the latter containing high amounts of viscous fiber and resistant starches. The HND diet incorporates features of other dietary interventions, but is designed to create advantages from multiple mechanisms, including the effect that high micronutrient food has in reducing cravings and overeating, and on lowering oxidative stress [8] and deposition of advanced glycation end products [9,10].

The HND diet is a plant-rich diet differing from other plant-based diets in some subtle, but significant, ways. Foods are rated based on total micronutrient content per calorie, which emphasizes consumption of greens and other non-starchy vegetables, such as onions, mushrooms, eggplant, peppers, tomatoes, and cauliflower, in unlimited quantity. High glycemic, high carbohydrate foods are reduced, while beans, peas, squash and intact grains are permitted. Nuts and seeds are the primary source of fat, while animal products are limited to 10 percent of calories or less. Basic recommendations include:

1) At least one large green salad a day, with inclusion of a nut/seed derived salad dressing.

2) One bowl of vegetable-bean soup daily.

3) 1 - 2 ounces of raw seeds and nuts daily (usually in salad dressing recipe).

4) Approximately 3 - 4 fresh fruits per day.

5) One large serving of steamed or stewed greens, with mushrooms, onions and other low-starch veggies.

6) Only one serving a day of non-bean starch, such as squash, steel cut oats, brown/wild rice.

7) Exclusion of white flour, sweets, and oils, while limiting animal products to 12 ounces per week.

The Mediterranean diet, which has been shown to reduce the risk of type 2 diabetes, encourages moderate amounts of fish and dairy, including fat and non-fat varieties, and emphasizes whole grains and extra virgin olive oil [11-13]. The HND diet, in contrast, suggests only small amounts of fish, non-fat dairy [14], whole grains and minimal amounts or no oil. The HND diet encourages more calories derived from vegetables and beans, as well as the intake of a moderate amount of fats from sources, such as nuts, which contain a combination of protein, fiber, phytonutrients, antioxidants and omega 3 fatty acids [15]. Tree nuts and peanut butter reduce the risk of developing diabetes in women [16,17]. Nuts significantly reduce the risk of coronary heart disease (CHD) and the risk of death from CHD [18-22] in type 2 diabetes patients.

The combination of the plant-based micronutrients recommended in the HND diet has the potential to improve results over those obtained in other medical nutrition studies. To provide an initial evaluation of the potential efficacy of the HND diet in participants with type 2 diabetes and to provide pilot data for large randomized clinical trials of the HND diet, we report a retrospective case series examining multiple parameters in 13 participants with type 2 diabetes, both before and after initiation of the HND diet.

2. METHODS

There were multiple inclusion criteria for this retrospective case series. The cases were selected based on two main criteria. First they needed to have a diagnosis of type 2 diabetes with documented baseline HbA1C readings before starting the HND diet. Second, the participants had to participate in phone interviews tracking their ongoing diet and historical dietary recall. As a result of these phone interviews, documented compliance with the dietary intervention of ≥90% was required for inclusion. Greater than 90% compliance was defined as

≤2 meals per week inconsistent with the HND diet and this minimum standard of consistency was necessary during the entire period of result tracking. The participants were not told of the compliance as an inclusion criterion until after analysis of their dietary intake was completed. Selection also required participants to fall into one of the following two categories during the pre-intervention period: they had a HbA1C > 7.0% with or without diabetes medications (n = 9); or they had a HbA1C > 6.0% with diabetes medications (n = 4). The participants were from two sources, Dr. Fuhrman's practice or Dr. Fuhrman's interactive website.

Dr. Fuhrman was not the primary care physician for these participants, but rather a specialist with expertise in medical nutrition, who contributed this dietary protocol advice to the participants. The office-based participants had an hour-long initial visit with Dr. Fuhrman, prior to starting the HND diet, and then had several 30-minute follow-up consultations. The web-based participants started the diet by reading the book *Eat to Live* and by accessing online support from the interactive website DrFuhrman.com, which provides web-based forums, recipes, and further information. Both the office-based participants and web-based participants had either visits or forum postings between 8/2007-8/2009. Data were collected and analyzed in 2009.

Ninety-seven charts and web postings from this two-year period were reviewed for eligibility. Fifty-two of these met baseline HbA1C eligibility requirements. Of these, 27 were available for phone interviews. Thirteen of these met dietary compliance eligibility criteria and were included in the study. Of these, 7 were office-based and 6 were web-based. All the participants were required to have copies of lab results sent by clinical laboratories. Participants' printed laboratory reports were collected from the charts for the office-based participants or were faxed/mailed by the participants or directly from the primary care physicians' offices for the web-based participants. For the web-based participants, biometric indices (weight, height and blood pressure) were measured at their primary care physicians' offices. For the office-based participants, the biometric parameters were measured at each visit by Dr. Fuhrman. Medication changes for the web-based participants were performed by their primary care physician. For the office-based participants, Dr. Fuhrman made the medication decisions.

This retrospective human subject analysis was reviewed and approved by the University of Pennsylvania's Institutional Review Board.

Descriptive analysis was performed for the participant characteristics using mean and standard deviation (SD) for continuous variables and proportion for categorical variables. The change of parameters over time after the start of the HND diet was plotted for each individual participant. For statistical comparison, the mean parameters measured before and at the last time point after starting the HND diet were calculated and compared using both the absolute change and percentage change. *p*-Values for testing whether absolute change and percentage change statistically differs from zero were determined using one-sample t-test. The correction for multiple statistical testing of many parameters was not considered as this study is a small pilot investigation. *p*-Value ≤ 0.05 was considered to be significant. For a participant with missing data in a parameter, the participant was excluded from the statistical comparison of this parameter, but was still included in the analysis of other parameters with complete data. The data analyses were performed using SAS v9.1 (SAS Institute Inc., Cary, NC).

3. RESULTS

Multiple baseline characteristics of each participant are illustrated (**Table 1**). The majority (69%) of participants was female. The demographics include 11 Cauca-

sians and 2 African-Americans. The mean age was 57 years old, ranging from 30 to 80 years old. BMI at baseline ranged from 25 to 45.6 kg/m^2. The mean HbA1C at baseline was 8.2%. Seventy-seven percent of the participants had hypertension (≥130/80 mmHg; based on ADA [23] and JNC7 [24] guidelines) and 92% had hyperlipidemia (based on the NCEP III guidelines [25]) before the HND diet. Sixty-two percent of participants had a family history of heart disease. The median length of follow-up with complete laboratory result time-points was 7 months (range: 5 to 42 months). During baseline and follow-up, a median of 3 laboratory result time-points (range: 2 to 8) per participant were obtained, with 92% having ≥3 laboratory result time-points. Most of the participants are/ were on the diet for much longer than the median follow-up period, though they did not have laboratory result time-points during this extended period.

After participants were on the HND diet for a median length of 7 months, most of the parameters showed significant improvements relative to pre-intervention levels (**Table 2**). The mean HbA1C dropped from 8.2% to

Table 1. Characteristics of participants at pre-intervention.

Pts	Sex	Age	Mo since Dx DM	HbA1C (%)	BMI (kg/m^2)	# meds	# DM meds	SBP (mm Hg) for pts with HTN	DBP (mm Hg) for pts with HTN	HDL (mg/dL)	Chol/HDL	Trig (mg/dL)
1	F	56	1	9.6	42.4	8	2	158	77	35	6.3	174
2	F	47	84	12.2	32.3	NA	NA	150	110	36	7.8	260
3	F	66	120	7.3	28.9	2	1	NA	NA	46	5.9	368
4	F	60	24	7.5	45.6	NA	NA	150	90	49	4.1	76
5	F	80	252	7.3	28.7	4	4	172	82	60	4	136
6	F	54	240	6.5	42.3	7	3	NA	NA	38	4	232
7	F	57	84	6.3	41.2	5	4	110	80	35	3.2	147
8	F	49	24	6.3	27.8	8	1	NA	NA	62	2.7	90
9	F	68	18	7.6	31.6	3	NA	160	90	59	4.9	190
10	M	30	12	10.7	32.0	1	1	150	90	48	6.1	102
11	M	74	84	7.6	25.5	3	1	158	75	63	2.4	102
12	M	39	84	10.4	43.3	2	2	145	90	NA	NA	NA
13	M	56	84	6.7	25.0	4	2	125	85	NA	NA	NA
Mean		57	85.0	8.15	34.3	4.3	2.1	148	87	48	4.7	171
SD		13.7	80.3	1.92	7.47	2.5	1.2	18	10	11	1.7	88
Mdn		56	84.0	7.50	32.0	4.0	2.0	150	88	48	4.1	147

[a]pts = patients; Mo since Dx DM = months since diagnosed with type 2 diabetes; # meds = number of overall medications; # DM meds = number of diabetes medications; SBP for pts with HTN = systolic blood pressure for participants with hypertension; DBP for pts with HTN = diastolic blood pressure for participants with hypertension; chol/HDL = cholesterol to HDL ratio; Trig = triglycerides; Total Chol = total cholesterol; Mdn = median; [b]NA = not applicable; NA = not available for lipids.

Table 2. A comparison of pre- and post-HND diet intervention parameters.

Parameters (# participants available for analysis)	Pre-intervention Mean (SE)	Post-intervention Mean (SE)	Change from baseline Mean (SE)	p-Value[***]	Percent change from baseline Mean (SE)	p-Value[***]
HbA1C (n = 13)	8.15 (0.53)	5.80 (0.15)	−2.35 (0.58)	0.002	25.4 (4.84)	0.0002
BMI (n = 13)	34.4 (2.07)	26.8 (1.72)	−7.79 (1.28)	<0.0001	−21.8 (2.56)	<0.0001
SBP (n = 10)	148 (5.70)	121 (4.72)	−25.8 (4.37)	0.0004	−17.2 (2.61)	0.0002
DBP (n = 10)	87 (3.14)	73.7 (1.53)	−12.9 (3.92)	0.01	−13.9 (3.57)	0.005
Chol/HDL ratio (n = 11)	4.67 (0.51)	3.62 (0.27)	−1.03 (0.50)	0.07	−13.9 (9.98)	0.19
Triglycerides (n = 11)	171 (26.6)	103 (11.2)	−69.2 (24.7)	0.02	−30.8 (11.0)	0.02
Total cholesterol (n = 11)	217 (19.0)	188 (11.8)	−21.2 (18.2)	0.27	−4.19 (8.86)	0.65
Weight (n = 13)	217 (15.4)	173 (13.8)	−47.0 (7.69)	<0.0001	−21.0 (2.66)	<0.0001
HDL (n = 11)	48.3 (3.40)	54.6 (4.80)	7.40 (2.93)	0.03	15.9 (6.16)	0.03
LDL (n = 11)	135 (17.7)	113 (8.64)	−15.7 (15.1)	0.33	2.8 (14.7)	0.85
Overall Meds (n = 11[*])	4.27 (0.74)	1.36 (0.36)	−2.91 (0.59)	0.0006	−67.1 (7.72)	<0.0001
Diabetes Meds (n = 10[*])	2.10 (0.38)	0.30 (0.15)	−1.80 (0.44)	0.003	−80 (11.1)	<0.0001
Hypertension Meds (n = 5[*])	1.80 (0.37)	0.60 (0.25)	−1.20 (0.37)	0.03	−63.3 (18.6)	0.03
Lipid Meds (n = 4[*])	1.25 (0.25)	0.50 (0.50)	−0.75 (0.25)	0.06	−75 (25.0)	0.06

[*]Restricted to those who were on study medications in pre-intervention; [**]Based on the last follow-up visit with data available; [***]From one-sample t-test whether the change from pre-intervention is statistically significant from 0.

5.8%, a 30% relative reduction that reached statistical significance (p = 0.002). The mean systolic blood pressure (SBP) decreased from 148 mmHg to 121 mmHg, with an 18% reduction from the pre-intervention period (p = 0.0004). Triglycerides decreased significantly from the pre-intervention period, with an absolute reduction of 67.2 mg/dl (p = 0.02) from a mean of 170.6 mg/dl to 103.4 mg/dl. Cholesterol/HDL ratio changed from 4.67 to 3.62 (p = 0.07). Of the 11 participants on medications, the mean number of drugs dropped from 4.3 to 1.4 (p = 0.0006) and 90% of participants on diabetes medications (n = 10) were able to completely discontinue or reduce their diabetes drug therapy. The one participant (ID = 11) who did not change diabetes medication was on the lowest starting dose of Glucophage XR 500 mg, once daily.

All of the participants (n = 13) had a decrease in HbA1C (**Figure 1(a)**). Sixty-two percent reached non-diabetic HbA1C levels of <6.0% at the last data point for the HND diet. There was a substantial and rapid reduction in mean HbA1C at 1 - 4 months (n = 11) on the HND diet (8.15% at baseline, 6.52% at 1 - 4 months, p = 0.02), and it declined further, reaching normoglycemic levels, to a mean HbA1C 5.95% (p = 0.006 as compared to baseline) at 5 - 9 months (n = 11). Three participants (ID = 1, 4, 12) had HbA1C data substantially beyond this

time period. One of the participants (ID = 1) started with glycosylated hemoglobin of 9.6%, reached a non-diabetic HbA1C of 5.4% at 15 months, and declined even further at 42 months to 4.8%, the participant's last lab results. The second participant (ID = 4) initially had a HbA1C of 7.5%, which approached near normoglycemic levels of 6.2% at the last time point of 18 months. The HbA1C of the third participant (ID = 12) dropped substantially from 7.6% to a non-diabetic level of 5.9% at the last data point of 34 months.

Every participant (n = 13) showed a reduction in BMI (**Figure 1(b)**). Forty-six percent of participants reached a normal BMI (<25 kg/m[2]) [26] at their last data point. Five of the participants experienced an almost 10 kg/m[2] or greater drop in BMI.

Each hypertensive type 2 diabetes participant (n = 10) in the study experienced a reduction in their SBP (**Figure 1(c)**) and 80% had a decrease of ≥20 mmHg. Of these participants, 7 experienced the considerable reduction within six months of starting the HND diet. Three hypertensive type 2 diabetes participants (ID = 1, 4, 13) had a sustained decline in their SBP with data out to 42, 18 and 34 months, respectively. Overall, participants who were on anti-hypertensive medications (n = 5) had a mean reduction in hypertensive medications of 67%.

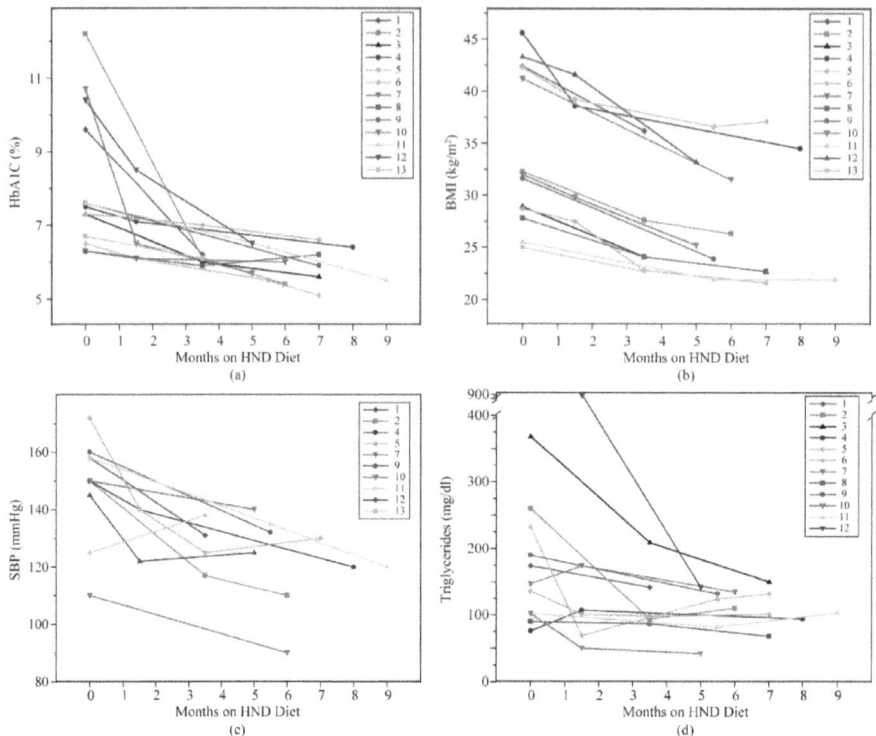

Figure 1. Graphs showing biometric data for each of the 13 study participants over time. Hemoglobin A1C (HbA1C; (a)), body mass index (BMI; (b)), systolic blood pressure (SBP; (c)) and triglycerides (d) are illustrated.

Most of the participants (n = 12) had a substantial drop in triglycerides within 6 months of starting the HND diet (**Figure 1(d)**). There were 11 participants who started the HND diet with dyslipidemia. Three participants (ID = 2, 3, 6) had triglycerides at pre-intervention that were >200 mg/dl. Their mean at baseline was 286 mg/dl with a precipitous mean reduction of 161 points. Another participant (ID = 12), whose pre-intervention levels were not obtained, had triglycerides of 885 mg/dl at 2 months which dropped to 142 mg/dl in 3 months, while still severely obese.

4. DISCUSSION

This case series of 13 type 2 diabetes participants demonstrated the mean reduction of 2.35% in the HbA1C, achieving statistical significance, with 62% reaching non-diabetic levels (HbA1C < 6.0%). Those with hyper-

tension reached a mean normotensive level.

Triglycerides were reduced while HDL was increased, both significantly. There was a substantial drop in the total number of drugs, and 90% of participants discontinued or decreased diabetes medications. None of these effects was due to hypoglycemic, hypertensive or lipid lowering medications, since there was no added or increased dose of medication in the study participants.

In addition to the substantial decrease in diabetes medications (n = 10) seen in this HND diet case series, 85% of participants (n = 11) were able to discontinue or reduce the dose of overall medications, including diabetes, hypertensive and lipid therapies. These participants were not nascent to diabetes, but had a mean disease duration of 7.1 years prior to the HND diet. The overall number of medications was reduced by 67%.

Although there are no head-to-head comparisons with other plant-based diets in type 2 diabetes patients, this study provides an initial assessment of the HND diet's effectiveness for diabetes. In several studies, it has been demonstrated that with a low fat vegan diet, type 2 diabetes could be better controlled than with the ADA diet [27,28]. In a randomized clinical trial contrasting a low fat vegan diet with the ADA diet, 43% of patients in the low fat vegan arm and 26% of patients in the ADA arm had a reduction in diabetes medications. Also, the HbA1C was reduced by a mean of 0.96% in 49 patients in the low fat vegan arm, and in the ADA arm, HbA1C was reduced by a mean of 0.56% in 50 patients [27].

Since there was a selection bias introduced into our study based on participant choice to participate on Dr. Fuhrman's website and/or office visits with Dr. Fuhrman, an accurate comparison of diet programs would best be accomplished by head-to-head analysis in a randomized prospective trial. However, the magnitude of effect of the HND diet in this case series indicates that the HND diet can be very effective in some participants.

Prior to starting the HND diet, 9 participants experienced diabetes-related complications and/or symptoms, including peripheral neuropathy in five participants, hypoglycemic episodes, cerebrovascular attack (CVA) or transient ischemic attack (TIA), and lethargy. All of the participants reported a reduction or complete dissipation of these symptoms. Further, none of the participants during the study period had any heart attacks, strokes, limb amputations, nephropathy or visual complaints.

Atherogenic dyslipidemia is a risk factor for heart disease [29]. Four of the participants in the HND diet case series (ID = 2, 3, 6, 12) had atherogenic dyslipidemia, which are triglycerides > 200 mg/dl and HDL < 50 mg/dl for a female or < 40 mg/dl for a male. After commencing the HND diet, all four of the participants' triglyceride levels were substantially reduced by over 100 points to 150 mg/dl or lower. The mean HDL rose 6.3 points to 54.6 mg/dl (n = 11), a statistically significant result compared to pre-HND diet levels ($p = 0.03$).

The CDC reports that 75% of type 2 diabetes patients also have hypertension, [30] of which only 36% are controlled [2]. The risk for cardiovascular disease begins to increase when blood pressure is > 115/75 mmHg. For every 20 mmHg increase in SBP and/or 10 mmHg increase in diastolic blood pressure, the risk for heart disease doubles [24]. Hypertensive type 2 diabetes participants (n = 10) in this HND diet case series showed a significant reduction in mean blood pressure from 148/87 mmHg to a normotensive level of 121/74 mmHg.

One potential mechanism for the decreases in glycemic levels, hypertension and hyperlipidemia in this HND diet case series is weight loss. However, the mean BMI at the last intervention point was 26.6 kg/m^2, which is considered overweight, yet the mean HbA1C reached a normoglycemic level of 5.8%. Six of the participants

whose BMIs decreased were still overweight or obese, yet 3 out of 6 reached normoglycemic levels (ID = 2, 6, 10). The remaining three (ID = 4, 7, 12) reached near normoglycemic levels. In fact, two of the participants (ID = 4 and 6) had BMIs at their last data points that are considered severely obese. Even participants (ID = 4, 6, 11, 13) who experienced either an increase or no change in BMIs (mean= +1.3%) between two data points demonstrated a decrease in HbA1C (mean= −6.8%) between these data points. Thus, the HND diet's beneficial effects on HbA1C appear to extend beyond weight loss.

In this case series, the HND diet has shown substantial sustainability and feasibility. The mean duration of the study with the 13 participants was 12.3 months. Of these participants, 62% were still on the diet at the study end point. Though five participants' HND diet compliance eventually lapsed, they all expressed interest in resuming, and four have been back on the diet for at least a few months. In terms of feasibility, 46% of the participants were able to garner knowledge about the HND diet for type 2 diabetes from the book *Eat to Live* and/or the supplemental interactive website. These six participants did not have a phone consult or office visit before initiating the diet or during the study period, though they could ask questions on the "ask the doctor" portion of the website. This is an indicator of the accessibility and clarity of the HND diet.

However, there are limitations to this study. It was a small retrospective case series with no control group. The study had selection bias, primarily because participants who reported their results on the website or chose to see Dr. Fuhrman in person may not represent the "typical" type 2 diabetes patient. In the study, 9 of 13 participants were female; its effectiveness in males needs further study. The HND diet may not work as effectively for everyone. For some, the HND diet may fail for numerous reasons, especially compliance. In this case series, participants were required to be at least 90% compliant with the diet. Of course, many patients also are not compliant with medications. To be successful, patients must have the proper knowledge and willpower. For the highly motivated individual, the HND diet appears to be an important weapon in the arsenal against type 2 diabetes.

5. CONCLUSION

This HND diet case series suggests benefits for patients with type 2 diabetes, its complications, and with some co-morbidities, such as heart disease risk, hypertension and hyperlipidemia. The HND diet may work well for some type 2 diabetes patients, but compliance with the HND diet may be an issue. This small case series has selection bias. However, the results of this study demonstrate that the HND diet can be a very effective intervention for some with type 2 diabetes. Therefore, further study is needed

REFERENCES

[1] Nathan, D.M., Buse, J.B., Davidson, M.B., Ferrannini, E., Holman, R.R., Sherwin, R. and Zinman, B. (2008) American diabetes association; European association for study of diabetes medical management of hyperglycemia in type 2 diabetes: A consensus algorithm for the initiation and adjustment of therapy. *Diabetes Care*, **32**, 193-203. doi:10.2337/dc08-9025

[2] Saydah, S.H., Fradkin, J. and Cowie, C. (2004) Poor control of risk factors for vascular disease among adults with previously diagnosed diabetes. *Journal of the American Medical Association*, **291**, 335-342. doi:10.1001/jama.291.3.335

[3] Montonen, J., Knekt, P., Härkänen, T., Järvinen, R., Heliövaara, M., Aromaa, A. and Reunanen, A. (2005) Dietary patterns and the incidence of type 2 diabetes. *American Journal of Epidemiology*, **161**, 219-227. doi:10.1093/aje/kwi039

[4] Ylönen, K., Alfthan, G., Groop, L., Saloranta, C., Aro, A., Virtanen, S.M. and the Botnia Research Group (2003) Dietary intakes and plasma concentrations of carotenoids and tocopherols in relation to glucose metabolism in subjects at high risk of type 2 diabetes: The Botnia dietary study. *American Journal of Clinical Nutrition*, **77**, 1434-1441.

[5] Jenkins, D.J., Kendall, C.W., Marchie, A., Jenkins, A.L., Augustin, L.S., Ludwig, D.S., Barnard, N.D. and Anderson J.W. (2003) Type 2 diabetes and the vegetarian diet. *American Journal of Clinical Nutrition*, **78**, 610S-616S.

[6] Bourn, D.M., Mann, J.I., McSkimming, B.J., Waldron, M.A. and Wishart, J.D. (1994) Impaired glucose tolerance and NIDDM: Does lifestyle intervention program have an effect? *Diabetes Care*, **17**, 1311-1319. doi:10.2337/diacare.17.11.1311

[7] Ford, E.S. and Mokdad, A.H. (2001) Fruit and vegetable consumption and diabetes mellitus incidence among US adults. *Preventive Medicine*, **32**, 33-39. doi:10.2337/diacare.17.11.1311

[8] Giammarioli, S., Filesi, C., Vitale, B., Cantagallo, A., Dragoni, F. and Sanzini, E. (2004) Effect of high intakes of fruit and vegetables on redox status in type 2 onset diabetes: A pilot study. *International Journal for Vitamin and Nutrition Research*, **74**, 313-320. doi:10.1024/0300-9831.74.5.313

[9] Vasdev, S., Gill, V. and Singal P. (2007) Role of advanced glycation end products in hypertension and atherosclerosis: Therapeutic implications. *Cell Biochemistry and Biophysics*, **49**, 48-63. doi:10.1007/s12013-007-0039-0

[10] Cervantes-Laurean, D., Schramm, D.D., Jacobson, E.L., Halaweish, I., Bruckner, G.G. and Boissonneault, G.A. (2006) Inhibition of advanced glycation end product formation on collagen by rutin and its metabolites. *Journal*

of Nutritional Biochemistry, **17**, 531-540. doi:10.1016/j.jnutbio.2005.10.002

[11] Benetou, V., Trichopoulou, A., Orfanos, P., Naska, A., Lagiou, P., Boffetta, P. and Trichopoulos, D. (2008) Conformity to traditional Mediterranean diet and cancer incidence: the Greek EPIC cohort. *British Journal of Cancer*, **99**, 191-195. doi:10.1038/sj.bjc.6604418

[12] Martinez-Gonzalez, M.A., de la Fuente-arrillaga, C., Nunez-Cordoba, J.M., Basterra-Gortari, F.J., Beunza, J.J., Vazquez, Z., Benito, S., Tortosa, A. and Bes-Rastrollo, M. (2008) Adherence to Mediterranean diet and risk of developing diabetes: Prospective cohort study. *British Medical Journal*, **336**, 1348-1351. doi:10.1136/bmj.39561.501007.BE

[13] Trichopoulou, A. and Lagiou, P. (2007) Healthy traditional Mediterranean diet: An expression of culture, history, and lifestyle. *Nutrition Reviews*, **55**, 383-389. doi:10.1111/j.1753-4887.1997.tb01578.x

[14] Lanou, A.J. (2009) Should dairy be recommended as part of a healthy vegetarian diet? Counterpoint. *American Journal of Clinical Nutrition*, **89**, 1638S-1642S. doi:10.3945/ajcn.2009.26736P

[15] Kris-Etherton, P.M., Hu, F.B., Ros, E. and Sabaté J. (2008) The role of tree nuts and peanuts in prevention of coronary heart disease. *Journal of Nutrition*, **138**, 1746S-1751S.

[16] Jiang, R., Manson, J.E., Sampfer, M.J., Liu, S., Willett, W.C. and Hu, F.B. (2002) Nut and peanut butter consumption and risk of type 2 diabetes in women. *Journal of the American Medical Association*, **288**, 2554-2560. doi:10.1001/jama.288.20.2554

[17] Sabate, J. and Ang, Y. (2009) Nuts and health outcomes: New epidemiologic evidence. *American Journal of Clinical Nutrition*, **89**, 1643S-1648S. doi:10.3945/ajcn.2009.26736Q

[18] Albert, C.M., Gaziano, J.M., Willett, W.C. and Manson, J.E. (2002) Nut consumption and decreased risk of sudden cardiac death in the Physicians' Health Study. *Archives of Internal Medicine*, **162**, 1382-1387.

[19] Hu, F.B., Stampfer, M.J., Manson, J.E., Rimm, E.B., Colditz, G.A., Rosner, B.A., Speizer, F.E., Hennekens, C.H. and Willett, W.C. (1998) Frequent nut consumption and risk of coronary heart disease in women: Prospective cohort study. *British Medical Journal*, **317**, 1341-1345. doi:10.1136/bmj.317.7169.1341

[20] Sabate, J. (1999) Nut consumption, vegetarian diets, ischemic heart disease risk and all-cause mortality: Evidence from epidemiologic studies. *American Journal of Clinical Nutrition*, **70**, 500S-503S.

[21] Li, T.Y., Brennan, A.M., Weddick, N.M., Mantzoros, C., Rifai, N. and Hu, F.B. (2009) Regular consumption of nuts is associated with a lower risk of cardiovascular disease in women with Type 2 Diabetes. *Journal of Nutrition*, **139**, 1333-1338. doi:10.3945/jn.108.103622

[22] Jenkins, D.J., Hu, F.B., Tapsell, L.C., Josse, A.R. and Kendall, C.W. (2008) Possible benefit of nuts in Type 2 diabetes. *Journal of Nutrition*, **138**, 1752S-1756S.

[23] American Diabetes Association (2008) Standards of medi-

cal care in diabetes-2008. *Diabetes Care*, **31**, S12-S54. doi:10.2337/dc08-S012

[24] Chobanian, A., Bakris, G., Black, H.R., Cushman, W.C., Green, L.A., Izzo, J.L. Jr., Jones, D.W., Materson, B.J., Oparil, S, Wright, J.T., Jr., Roccella, E.J. and the National High Blood Pressure Education Program Coordinating Committee (2003) The Seventh Report of the Joint National Committee on Prevention, Detection, Evaluation, and Treatment of High Blood Pressure. *Journal of the American Medical Association*, **289**, 2560-2571. doi:10.1001/jama.289.19.2560

[25] Expert Panel on Detection, Evaluation and Treatment of High Blood Cholesterol in Adults (2001) Executive summary of the third report of the national cholesterol education program (NCEP) expert panel on detection, evaluation, and treatment of high blood cholesterol in adults (adult treatment panel III). *Journal of the American Medical Association*, **285**, 2486-2497. doi:10.1001/jama.285.19.2486

[26] Classification of overweight and obesity by BMI, waist circumference, and associated diseaserRisks (2009) http://www.nhlbi.nih.gov/health/public/heart/obesity/lose_wt/bmi_dis.htm

[27] Barnard, N.D., Cohen, J., Jenkins, D.J., Turner-McGrievy, G., Gloede, L., Jaster, B., Seidl, K., Green, A.A. and Talpers, S. (2006) A low-fat vegan diet improves glycemic control and cardiovascular risk factors in a randomized clinical trial in individuals with type 2 diabetes. *Diabetes Care*, **29**, 1777-1783. doi:10.2337/dc06-0606

[28] Barnard, N.D., Cohen, J., Jenkins, D.J., Turner-McGrievy, G., Gloede, L., Green, A. and Ferdowsian, H. (2009) A low-fat vegan diet and a conventional diabetes diet in the treatment of type 2 diabetes: A randomized, controlled, 74-wk clinical trial. *American Journal of Clinical Nutrition*, **89**, 1588S-1596S. doi:10.3945/ajcn.2009.26736H

[29] Arca, M., Montali, A., Valiante, S., Campagna, F., Pigna, G., Paoletti, V., Antonini, R., Barilla, F., Tanilli, G., Vestri, A. and Gaudio, C. (2007) Usefulness of atherogenic dyslipidemia for predicting cardiovascular risk in patients with angiographically defined coronary artery disease. *American Journal of Cardiology*, **100**, 1511-1516. doi:10.1016/j.amjcard.2007.06.049

[30] National Diabetes Statistics 2007 (2008) Internet accessed 25 May 2009. http://www.diabetes.niddk.nih.gov/DM/PUBS/statistics/

THE AMAZING NATHAN PRITIKIN
(1915-1985)

Before Dr. Dean Ornish published his heart disease reversal with diet, exercise, and meditation in Lancer in 1990 and Dr. Esselstyne reversed heart disease with diet and drugs, there was Nathan Pritikin, an engineer, who in World War II designed the optics for the Nordon Bombsight. When he was diagnosed with heart disease in his 40's, he was not willing to except the fatalistic prognoses and did his own research. He studied the diet of cultures around the world particularly Uganda. He finally arrived at a plant based diet dropping his cholesterol from 280 down to 94 reversing his own heart disease before doing the same for thousands of others in his lifestyle clinics and books. Before he lost his 28-year battle with radiation-induced cancer and took his own life. He left instruction for his autopsy to be revealed because he wanted to show the world what his diet could do. The autopsy findings were published in the New England Journal of Medicine 30 years after his original heart disease diagnosis which was considered incurable at the time. His coronary arteries were soft and pliable widely patent throughout. In a man 69 years old, the near absence of atherosclerosis and the complete absence of its effects are remarkable. Pitkin's life's work continued through his research foundation, switching its focus from heart disease to cancer.

Senator George McGovern was chairman of the special select committee on nutrition and human needs. After reading their goals for changing the American diet I wondered if McGovern knew Pritikin. Not only did they know each other they we're close friends. Senator McGovern gave the eulogy at Mr. Pritikin's funeral. The McGovern committee suffered the usual institutional limitations of select committees, in that they could highlight problems but could not report legislation to the floor.

In January 1977, after having held hearings on the national diet, the McGovern committee issued a new set of nutritional guidelines for Americans that sought to combat leading killer conditions such as heart disease, certain cancers, stroke, high blood pressure, obesity, diabetes, and arteriosclerosis. Titled "Dietary Goals for the United States," but also known as the "McGovern Report", they suggested that Americans eat less fat, less cholesterol, less refined and processed sugars, and more complex carbohydrates and fiber. (Indeed, it was the McGovern report that first used the term complex carbohydrate, denoting "fruit, vegetables and whole-grains." The recommended way of accomplishing this was to eat more fruits, vegetables, and whole grains, and less high-fat meat, egg, and dairy products. While many public health officials had said all of this for some time, the committee's issuance of the guidelines gave it higher public profile.

The committee's "eat less" recommendations triggered strong negative reactions from the cattle, dairy, egg and sugar industries, including from McGovern's home state. The American Medical Association protested as well, reflecting its long espoused belief that people should see their doctor for individual advice rather than follow guidance for the public as a whole. Some scientists also thought the committee's conclusions needed further expert review. Others felt that the job of promulgating recommendations belonged to the Food and Nutrition Board of the National Research Council. Under heavy pressure, the committee held further hearings, and issued a revised set of guidelines in late 1977 which adjusted some of the advice regarding salt and cholesterol and watered down the wording regarding meat consumption.

Senator McGovern was a B24 bomber pilot during World War II flying 35 combat missions over German occupied Europe. He was awarded several air medals including the Distinguished Flying Cross. His bomber used the Nordon Bombsight. Senator McGovern died in 2012 at age 90

HEART DISEASE

Heart Disease is the number one cause of death for diabetics and the number one cause of death for men and women in America. About every minute an American has a heart attack.

The buildup of plaque, known as atherosclerosis, is the hardening of the arteries by pockets of cholesterol-rich gunk that builds up within the inner linings of the blood vessels. This process occurs over decades, slowly bulging into the space inside the arteries, narrowing the path for blood to flow. The restriction of blood circulation to the heart muscle can lead to chest pain and pressure, known as angina when people try to exert themselves. If the plaque ruptures, a blood clot can form within the artery. This sudden blockage of blood flow can cause a heart attack, damaging or even killing part of the heart.

When you think about heart disease, you may think of friends or loved ones who suffered for years with chest pain and shortness of breath before they finally succumbed. However, for the majority of Americans who die suddenly from heart disease, the very first symptom may be their last. It's called "sudden cardiac death." This is when death occurs within an hour of symptom onset. In other words, you may not even realize you're at risk until it's too late. You could be feeling perfectly fine having dinner with family and friends and then an hour later, you're gone forever.

Atherosclerosis is also the number one cause of disability in America; angina, lower back pain, erectile dysfunction (40 percent of American men over 40 have E.D. which should stand for early death). Men with E.D. should be considered at cardiac risk until proven otherwise.

HEART DISEASE STARTS IN CHILDHOOD

In 1953, a study published in the Journal of the American Medical Association changed the understanding of the development of heart disease. Researchers conducted a series of three hundred autopsies on American casualties of the Korean War, with an average age of around twenty-two. Shockingly, 77 percent of soldiers already had visible evidence of coronary atherosclerosis. Some even had arteries that were blocked off 90 percent or more. The study "dramatically showed that atherosclerotic changes appear in the coronary arteries years and decades before the age at which coronary heart disease (CHD) becomes a clinically recognized problem."

Later studies of accidental death victims between the ages of three and twenty-six found that fatty streaks—the first stage of atherosclerosis—were found in nearly all American children by age ten. By the time, we reach our twenties and thirties, these fatty streaks can turn into full-blown plaques like those seen in the young American GIs of the Korean War. And by the time we're forty or fifty they can start killing us off.

The question isn't whether or not you want to eat healthier to prevent heart disease but whether or not you want to eat healthier to reverse the heart disease you very likely already have.

The current official recommendation is to have a total cholesterol under 200. Over 240 is considered high, 200 to 239 borderline high, so under 200 is desirable. So you would imagine that the average cholesterol of people who have heart attacks would be 250...300 somewhere in the high range. A major study was published in 2011 by the American Heart Journal, 65,000 people hospitalized with acute coronary syndromes, like myocardial infarctions-heart attacks, across 344 hospitals. What was their average cholesterol on admission? 170! If you saw your doctor and maybe you have some concerns family history, your diet not that great, your neighbor just had a heart attack etc. and your cholesterol came back 170 well within the "desirable range," your doctor would tell you to keep up the good work and send you on your merry way. Based on this data maybe the next time you see him is when you arrive in an ambulance if you're lucky enough to make it that far. Most people admitted to hospitals with heart attacks have "normal" cholesterols. Having a "normal" cholesterol in a society where it's "normal" to drop dead of heart disease, is not necessarily a good thing. Desirable cholesterol levels leave a lot to be desired.

According to William C. Roberts, the editor in chief of the American Journal of Cardiology, the only critical risk factor for atherosclerotic plaque buildup is cholesterol, specifically elevated LDL cholesterol in your blood. LDL is called bad cholesterol, because it's the vehicle by which cholesterol is deposited into your arteries. Autopsies of thousands of young accident victims have shown that the level of cholesterol in the blood was closely correlated with the amount of atherosclerosis in their arteries. To drastically reduce LDL cholesterol levels, you need to drastically reduce your intake of three things: trans fat, which comes from processed foods and naturally from meat and dairy; saturated fat, found mainly in animal product and junk foods; and to a lesser extent dietary cholesterol, found exclusively in animal-derived foods, especially eggs. (Roberts, 2009)

IT'S THE CHOLESTEROL, STUPID!

Dr. Roberts hasn't only been editor in chief of the American Journal of cardiology for more than thirty years; he's the executive director of the Baylor Heart and Vascular Institute and has authored more than a thousand scientific publications and written more than a dozen textbooks on cardiology. He knows his stuff.

In his editorial "It's the Cholesterol, Stupid!" Dr. Roberts argued (as noted earlier) that there is only one true risk factor for coronary heart disease: cholesterol. You could be an obese, diabetic, smoking couch potato and still not develop atherosclerosis, he argues, as long as the cholesterol level in your blood is low enough.

The optimal LDL cholesterol level is probably 50 or 70 mg/dL, and apparently, the lower, the better. That's where you start out at birth, that's the level seen in populations largely free of heart disease, and that's the level at which the progression of atherosclerosis appears to stop in cholesterol-lowering trials. An LDL around 70md/dL corresponds to a total cholesterol level reading of about 150, the level below which no deaths from coronary heart disease were reported in the famous Framingham Heart Study, a generations-long project to identify risk factors for heart disease. The population target should therefore be a total cholesterol level under 150mg/dL. "If such a goal was created," Dr. Roberts wrote, "the great scourge of the Western world would be essentially eliminated."

The average cholesterol for people living in the United States is much higher than 150 mg/dL; it hovers around 200mg/dL.

To become virtually heart-attack proof, you need your LDL cholesterol at least under 70 mg/dL. Dr. Roberts noted that there are only two ways to achieve this for our population: to put more than a hundred million Americans on a lifetime of medications or to recommend they all eat a diet centered around whole plant foods.

All health plans cover cholesterol-lowering statin drugs, so why change your diet if you can simply pop a pill every day for the rest of your life? Unfortunately, these drugs don't work nearly as well as people think, and they may cause undesirable side effects. (Roberts, 2009)

For individuals at high risk for heart disease who are unwilling or unable to bring down their cholesterol levels naturally with dietary changes, the benefits of statins generally outweigh the risks.

Potential for liver or muscle damage, the reason some doctors routinely order regular blood tests for patients on these drugs, is to monitor for liver toxicity. Test also the blood for muscle breakdown products, but biopsies reveal that people on statins can show evidence of muscle damage even if their blood work is normal and they exhibit no symptoms of muscle soreness or weakness. The decline in muscular strength and performance sometimes associated with these drugs may not be a big deal for younger individuals, but they can place our seniors at increased risk for falls and injury.

Recently, concerns have been raised. As I mentioned earlier, in 2012, the U.S. Food and Drug Administration announced newly mandated safety labeling on statin drugs to warn doctors and patients about their potential for brain-related side effects, such as memory loss and confusion. Statin drugs also appeared to increase the risk of developing diabetes. In 2013, a study of several thousand breast cancer patients reported that long-term use of statins may as much double a woman's risk of invasive breast cancer. The primary killer of women is heart disease, not cancer, so the benefits of statins may still outweigh the risks, but why accept any risk at all if you can lower your cholesterol naturally. (FDA, 2012)

Until Recently, The American Diabetes Association (ADA) recommended that people with diabetes aim for LDL levels less than 100 mg/dL. For people with diabetes who also have cardiovascular disease, the (ADA) recommended lowering LDL to less than 70mg/dL. Here's the big news: Last year, the ADA recommended a statin-type cholesterol-lowering drug for most people with diabetes, no matter their LDL cholesterol levels.

Whether you're at moderate or high risk for cardiovascular disease determines the particular statin drug and dose for you. The ADA recommends other cholesterol lowering medications only if you don't tolerate a statin medication or otherwise don't benefit from it.

The ADA-like the American Heart Association (AHA)- no longer has specific targets for LDL cholesterol. However, both the National Lipid Association (NLA) and the American Association of Clinical Endocrinologists (AACE) recommend LDL goals of less than 70mg/dL for people with diabetes at high risk for heart trouble and less than 100 mg/dl for others.

All Four Organizations Agree: A Statin is The First Drug of Choice.

Both the ADA and AHA changed their recommendations on statin drugs, says Evan Sisson, Pharm. D, CDE associate professor at Virginian Commonwealth University School of Pharmacy and a spokesperson for the American Association of Diabetes Educators.

We need to prevent some of those 600,000 deaths each year. Statins do that, Sisson says. "They protect against heart attacks."

Not only do statin drugs lower LDL cholesterol levels, they appear to have an anti-inflammatory effect and stabilize plaque in the blood vessels, says James Underberg M.D. FACPM, FACP, FNLA, clinical lipidologist and an executive committee member of the NLA.

When plaque ruptures and spews inflammatory contents inside a vessel and an obstructing blood clot forms on that rupture, blocking blood flow, you have a greater risk of heart attack or stroke.

In most situations, the ADA doesn't recommend combining a statin drug with another cholesterol-lowering medication to further reduce LDL levels. The proof of benefit relative to the risk of side effects is not there, they say.

But because the NLA and AACE recommend specific LDL goals, they support combining medications to bring patients' cholesterol numbers to target.

New Meds on the horizon, a brand new class of cholesterol lowering medications, will soon be available, and they differ from current therapy in many ways.

The don't come in a bottle. You don't swallow a pill every day. Rather, a PCSK9 inhibitor is injected every other week or so.

Some people in clinical trials have seen LDL cholesterol plummet to levels well below 40mg/dL even in people who have already benefited from a statin drug, Underberg says.

But it will take more studies to show that these new drugs prevent heart attacks, he says.

Sisson says that PCSK9 inhibitors are currently indicated for a limited group of people:

- Patients with established heart disease who are unable to adequately reduce LDL cholesterol with current therapies.

- Individuals with a genetic condition called heterozygous familial hypercholesterolemia.

Sisson and Underberg say the new drug class appears to be safe, through it's only been tested on a small number of people. And they're pricey and may cost you or your insurance company $12,000 a year.

If your concerned about your LDL cholesterol dropping too low, Underberg says that individuals with genetically low LDL levels of less than 25 mg/dL do live healthy, active lives without heart disease.

In fact, PCSK9 inhibitors were developed after researchers learned of people who have genetically low cholesterol due to a gene mutation. PCSK9 inhibitors target that gene.

Plant-based diets have been shown to lower cholesterol just as effectively as first-line statin drugs, but without the risks. In fact, the "side effects" of healthy eating tend to be good – less cancer, reversed and prevent diabetes and protection of the liver and brain.

HEART DISEASE IS REVERSIBLE

Lifestyle medicine pioneers Nathan Pritikin, Dr. Dean Ornish, and Dr. Caldwell Esselstyn, Jr. took patients with advanced heart disease and put them on the kind of plant-based diet followed by Asian and African populations who didn't suffer from heart disease. Their hope was that a healthy enough diet would stop the disease process and keep it from progressing further.

But instead, something miraculous happened. Their patients' heart disease started to reverse. These patients were getting better. As soon as they stopped eating an artery-clogging diet, their bodies were able to start dissolving away some of the plaque that had built up. Arteries opened up without drugs or surgery, even in some cases of patients with severe triple-vessel heart disease. This suggests their bodies wanted to heal all along but were just never given the chance.

Dr. Michael Greger, M.D. says it's "the best kept secret in medicine." Given the right conditions, the body heals itself. Within about 15 years of stopping smoking, your lung cancer risk approaches that of a lifelong nonsmoker. Your lungs can clear out all that tar buildup and, eventually, it's almost as if you never smoked at all.

"Oxidized LDL levels is a better indicator of heart disease risk," states Dr. Barry Sears. So why don't physicians use oxidized LDL levels as an indicator of heart disease risk? First, the test is much more difficult to do than a simple cholesterol test. Second, it ruins a great story that is easy to communicate to the patient. Third, the best way of reducing oxidized LDL levels is natural anti-oxidants, such as polyphenols, that have no patent protection (3,4). Reducing oxidized LDL cholesterol requires having plenty of antioxidants in your diet with polyphenols the most powerful.

Another new entry into the LDL story. This is "super-sticky" LDL. This new type of LDL particle may be even worse than oxidized cholesterol in promoting the development of heart disease. This "super-sticky" LDL comes from the formation of advanced glycosylation end products (AGEs).

The best way to reduce the production of "super-sticky" LDL is to reduce blood sugar levels. This helps explain why individuals with diabetes are two to three times more likely to develop heart disease. The best way to reduce elevated blood sugar is the Zone diet. That's why the latest dietary recommendations for the treatment of diabetes by the Joslin Diabetes Research Center at Harvard Medical School are essentially identical to the Zone diet. This is Not true the best diet is the one I mention.

Researchers wanted to know what caused the inflammation from meat products. Was it the heme iron or animal fat maybe the protein possible the IGF-1. They used a sausage and Egg McMuffin. What was it that causes your entire artery tree and pulmonary system to become inflamed dead meat bacteria. Researchers found that boiling meat for 2 hours didn't kill the endotoxins nor did an acid bath of your digestive juices in your stomach and it takes about 5 to 6 hours for your body's defenses to return to normal just in time for lunch. A quarter pound of hamburger meat has 100 million bacteria.

Inflammation causes free radicals and salty meals suppress the superoxide dismutase which eliminate a million free radicals a second.

After stopping statins, I was concerned about lowering my cholesterol. Pritikin had taken a few years to bring his cholesterol down from 300 to 100 but that was 50 years a go and we've made exponential advancements since then. So I read Dr. Caldwell Esselstyn book. Who did Dr. Caldwell Esselstyn read before setting up his heart disease program at the Cleveland Clinic? Nathan Pritikin.

MY PHONY HEART ATTACK

I'm running on my treadmill about 10 minutes before I finish my run I get a sharp pain in the middle of my chest. It's intense but not unbearable, so I take a shower dress and head for my office. Pain is still there so I call my primary care doctor and get the nurse who is emphatic that I go to the emergency room. I'm close to the research and teaching hospital, the largest hospital in my state, so I pull in and park. I walked into the emergency room and they have a sign which reads "If you are having chest pains talk to this person" and it has an arrow pointing to a desk with a not particularly friendly lady. She calls a technician who leads me back to an examination room takes images and blood, when I belch embarrassingly loud, the pain seems to subside. I ask if everything looks ok and he said "didn't see anything and enzymes are normal" as he walks me into intensive care and said this is protocol. "You're going to keep me overnight?" "Yep, we're going to do more tests. It's cautionary." After several hours in ICU, they moved me to a private room.

This was a Friday and I had a date so I texted my lady friend that I'm in the hospital getting some tests. I'm fine but my cell phone battery is low so If I don't reply I'm not dead but my cell phone is. My night nurse asked me how I got my blood sugar down (she's diabetic) so I wrote out the diet and exercise and listed a couple of books. You get this, a nurse in a teaching hospital with a world recognized cancer center and maybe a 1000 doctors, is asking a securities trader how to treat her diabetes. I'm happy to help.

Saturday morning, young cardiologists start coming by to interview and examine me one at a time. By the time the 4th one came in with the same routine I explained "I have told this story 3 times. Go ask your colleagues." Then about 45 minutes later they all return with the head of the cardiology department, a distinguished older gentleman whose bald looks fit, and wearing an Armani suit.

He exams me, comments that I'm in pretty good shape and he agrees he doesn't think I had a heart attack but he wants me to stay over until Monday for an M.R.I. I told him I will come back but I'm not staying in the hospital. He asked if I had a defibrillator. I told him no, but I would pick up one on the way home (by the way you can get a used defibrillator for around $1200.00). Only the young female cardiologist was interested in Dr. Esselstyn program. The rest looked at me like I was speaking in Greek.

Sunday morning I'm with my fishing buddy headed for some mountain streams and explaining my experience and I start getting that chest pain again. Randy, who's always prepared reaches into his pocket and pulls out two lent covered tums. 10minutes later no pain.

I returned for my imaging and one of the technician who was diabetic asked me how I lowered my blood sugar. I asked for his email and later sent him the information (they see diabetic and my A1C in my medical records). The M.R.I. took about 25 minutes during which you lie on your back arms pointing away from your chest and the device spins around your chest. Another doctor, I'm not sure if he's a cardiologist or radiologist, examines the pictures on a monitor and after about 15 minutes standing behind him, I asked if my heart and coronary arteries are ok, and he says yes, fine. Well can I leave? You're finished? Yah. Sure!

When I told my friend, I lowered my LDL to 67. She said perfect, it will be easy for you to remember, I asked How's that? She said "it's the same as your IQ."

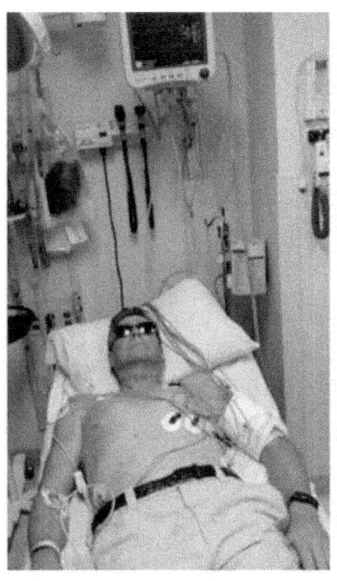
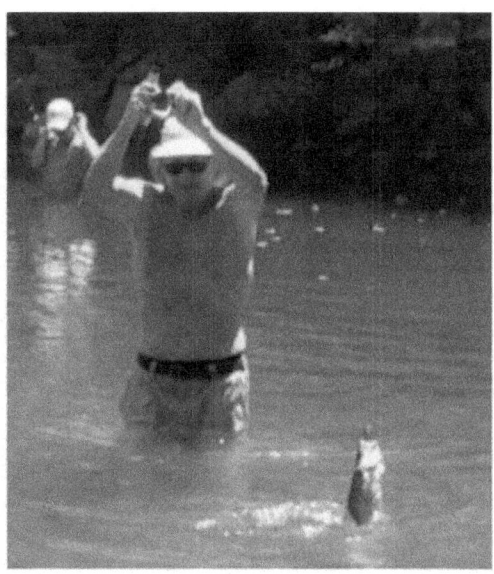

Before Tums   After Tums

CANCER

NEW BLOOD TEST FOR CANCER

The ONCOblot Test is a highly sensitive blood test for cancer. It confirms the presence of cancer as well as the tissue of origin through the detection of EMOX2 proteins. ENOX2 proteins are detected 4-10 years in advance of clinical symptoms.

The ENOX2 protein species in the blood is unique to malignant cells and absent from non-cancer cells. These proteins can be detected in early development. The ONCOblot test identifies the ENOX2 markers and the direct visualization of a marker presence significantly reduces false positives.

The ONCOblot test has filed it's 501 with the FDA for approval cost around $850.00

The ONCOblot test reveals the tissue of origin of the ENOX2 protein. The ONCOblot database contains the following 25+cancers:

Bladder	Leukemia	Pancreatic
Breast	Non-Small cell	Prostate
Cervical	Lung Small cell	Sarcoma
Endometrial	Lymphoma	Squamous Cell

Esophageal	Melanoma	Follicular Thyroid
Gastric	Mesothelloma	Papillary Thyroid
Hepatocelluar	Myelom	Testicular Germ Cell
Kidney	Ovarian	Uterine
Colorectal		

Evidence linking diabetes and high insulin levels to certain cancers has grown stronger over the past several years, leading scientists to investigate potential mechanisms. A growing body of evidence is finding that having diabetes or signs of insulin resistance may lead to an increased risk of certain cancers. The connection is strongest among certain types of cancers, including kidney, pancreatic and colorectal.

"The trend emerging [in this area] is that the type 2 diabetes associated with high insulin levels is the biggest problem relating to cancer risk," said, M.D., a professor at the Department of Oncology and Director of the Cancer Prevention Research Unit at McGill University. "But it's not just type 2 diabetes," he added, "this link is evident for everyone with prediabetes, which is a much larger group."

THE INSULIN-CANCER CONNECTION

According to the Centers for Disease Control and Prevention, approximately 90 million Americans are estimated to have prediabetes, a condition that increases the risk for developing diabetes. Hyperinsulinemia, too much insulin in the blood, is a sign of prediabetes. People can be unaware they have prediabetes for years before symptoms and rising glucose levels result in a diabetes diagnosis.

Hyperinsulinemia, type 2 diabetes and cancer all share a major risk factor: high body fat. AICR's second expert report found that high body fat is convincingly linked to increased risk of several cancers, including pancreatic and colorectal.

The hormonal changes spurred by high body fat may be leading to increased risk of cancer and type 2 diabetes. Hyperinsulinemia could also act independent of body fat to increase cancer risk. "We know that lots of tumors have insulin receptors and research suggests insulin plays an important role in cancer, but it does not have to be a direct link, "said Dr. Pollak. "There may be other areas that insulin could affect." Yet insulin, which stimulates cell proliferation and growth, appears to be one of the key mediators.

High levels of insulin, independent of body fat, are linked to increased production of insulin-like growth-factor 1 (IGF-1). And IGF-1, which shares a similar structure to insulin, play a key role in cell growth, proliferation and inhibiting apoptosis.

Dr. Joel Fuhrman restricts his patients to only six ounces of animal protein per week. The main reason is that, for many people with diabetes, even a relatively low amount of animal protein in the diet could raise a IGF-1.

There is a tremendous amount of evidence regarding the life-span enhancing effect of lower levels of IGF-1, especially in adulthood. Lower levels of IGF-1 are associated with enhanced insulin sensitivity and enhanced life span. The higher the biological value of the protein consumed, and the more of it consumed, the more IGF-1 produced. So the regular consumption of animal products is the most significant factor promoting IGF-1. Muscle tissue can produce its own IGF-1 in response to resistance exercise, but this does not raise systemic IGF-1 unless a diet that is rich in animal protein is consumed

IGF-1 AND CANCER

The largest concern about elevated IGF-1 from our modern diet is its link to cancer. Elevated hormone levels caused by the Western diet are thought to contribute to the high rates of cancer in the modern world not just sex hormones, such as estrogen and testosterone, but insulin and IGF-1 as well. The connection between increased IGF-1 signaling and cancer has been known for years—in fact, cancer drugs targeting the IGF-1 pathway began to be developed in the late 1990s, with over seventy clinical trials since then, many with encouraging results. Because IGF-1 signaling plays a key role in tumor growth, reducing IGF-1 signaling plays a key role in tumor growth, reducing IGF-1 levels by dietary methods is now considered by most scientists studying this subject to be an effective cancer-prevention measure. IGF-1 signaling is involved in a number of processes relevant to tumor growth: proliferation, adhesion, migration, invasion, angiogenesis, and metastatic growth. A diet that is rich in antioxidants and phytochemicals results in reduced inflammation, oxidative stress, and IGF-1, which are critical to protecting against cancer and maximizing longevity.

The composition of protein and the amount consumed also modify IGF-1 levels. Protein that is rich in the full array of essential amino acids causes larger increases in IGF-1 compared to protein not as biologically complete. Plant sources of protein are less concentrated. They supply adequate protein, but not excessive amounts like animal products do. For example, milk and dairy products contribute to this excessive IGF-1 in circulation. In a meta-analysis of eight randomized controlled trials, circulating IGF-1 was found to be higher in milk consuming groups compared to control groups.

Refined Carbohydrates promote IGF-1. Although protein is the most important determinant of IGF-1 levels, excess intake of refined carbohydrates can also have an effect. Insulin regulates energy metabolism and affects IGF-1 signaling by increasing production of IGF-1 and decreasing IGF-1- binding proteins. It is likely that the Western diet increases IGF-1 via both excess protein and excess refined carbohydrate. Type 2 diabetes is associated with breast, colon, and pancreatic cancers, and there is evidence that insulin -mediated stimulation of IGF-1 production is partially responsible. Recognize that refined carbohydrates from processed foods and our nation's preoccupation with eating animal protein are both at the core of our cancer and diabetes epidemic.

For many people, even a moderate amount of animal protein in the diet maintains unfavorably elevated IGF-1 levels and impedes the cholesterol-lowering and blood -sugar-lowering effects of a plant-based diet.

There is a rare genetic deficiency that leads to a type of dwarfism that's IGF-1 deficiency their growth factor one is so low they only grow about 3 ½ feet tall. But they almost never get Cancer. Their relatives who don't have this deficiency die of cancer at the same rate as the general public about 20%. The percentage of Little People dying of cancer Zero.

So researchers thought why not have the best of both worlds all the IGF-1 while we grow and when we reach adulthood keep your IGF level low.

Pritikin Institute did an elegant study that drew blood from 3 different groups and just dropped it on a petri dish filled with cancer cells and stood back and watched what happened. The first group were couch potatoes and ate the western diet their blood killed a few cancer cells. The second group the same diet but they had exercised an hour a day vigorously for 14 years their blood killed about 70% more than the couch potatoes. The third group was placed on a plant based diet and walked 30 minutes a day for only 12 days killed more cancer cells then the vigorous exercise group.

Subsequent studies showed exercise can reduce the IGF-1 but plant based diet increased the bodies binding protein (one way our body tries to protect itself from cancer by releasing a binding protein to tie up the IGF-1. A few weeks on a plant based diet cancer cell growth drops and cancer cell death shoots up.

A little more than 2% of all human cancer is attributable to purely genetic or congenital factors. The rest involved external factors such as our diets. The most comprehensive summary of evidence on diet and cancer ever compiled recommends we should eat mostly foods of plant origin to help prevent cancer not just eat whole grains, beans, vegetables, and fruit ever day but every meal.

On foods that may increase cancer risk these researchers didn't mince words for example don't minimize soda intake avoid it. Don't just cut back on bacon, ham, hot dogs, sausage, lunch meat, but avoid processed meat—period--because data do not show any level of intake that can confidently be shown not to be associated with risk.

Processed meat could be a powerful multi-organ carcinogen, but may increase the risk of heart disease and diabetes. Red meat was bad, but processed meat was worse and that included white meat like chicken and turkey slices. Processed meat consumption was associated with increased risk of death.

Colon cancer is the second leading cause of cancer death with American men and women after lung cancer. Researchers at the University of Pittsburg and the Royal college of London swapped diets with 20 African Americans who had colon cancer markers with 20 rural South Africans. Colon cancer is rare in Black South Africans. After two weeks the cancer markers had disappeared from the African Americans and appeared of the South Africans. Researchers said it was the 50 grams of restricted starch in the rural African diet.

But you have the same low rate of colon cancer in urban South Africans who are as inactive and overweight as Americans and eat processed food and still have that low rate of colon cancer they rarely eat meat.

Phytates in grains, nuts, seeds, and beans inhibit cancer cell migration in human colon cancer cells and human breast cancer cells.

The famous Irish surgeon, Dr. Denis Burkitt who discovered a childhood leukemia, but was famous for his theory on colon cancer. After 25 years in Africa not seeing one native African with colon cancer he concluded it was the fiber and possibly the native Africans squatting vs sitting to defecate. The American Cancer Society in a study using fruit, vegetable and beans concluded that the fruit and vegetables did not seem to reduce the risk of polyps but phytates in beans did--not the fiber.

Pritikin in the lost lectures explains eating the SDA diet produces 10 times the amount of bile to handle all the fat. This bile creates an environment that promotes anaerobic bacteria (don't require oxygen) that feed on the bile and multiply. The waste product from these little one cell creatures who live in our lower intestines rent free is deoxycholic acid and the hormone estrogen which passes back into the blood stream excess estrogen contributes to the risk of breast cancer and deoxycholic acid may be carcinogenic and it's being manufactured close to the colon.

Pritikin mentioned high cholesterol as a promoting factor in cancer. Dr. Standler of Chicago did a study 900 men all smokers he was trying to determine a relationship on how much they smoked and how long they smoked and who got cancer no relationship he checked other variables nothing. Then he checked their blood values those who had cholesterol below 225 had 5 cases of lung cancer per 1000 those with cholesterol 250 15 cases per thousand and those with cholesterol 275 had 37 cases per 1000. This was also demonstrated with animal studies by giving animals cancer tumors and adding cholesterol to their diet the tumors growth was increased add more cholesterol more growth.

Pritikin said the cholesterol paralyzed the big Macrophage white blood cell that eats cancer cells.

Dr. Wenders 1980 Head of American Health Foundation of New York testified in front of Senator McGovern's sub-committee that in this country if we could drop the amount of fat and cholesterol in the diet to the levels Pritikin recommended three primary cancers would disappear colon, breast, and prostate.

Pritikin also suggested that if we could lower the Pro Active Level in American women to that of the Japanese who had only 10% of the breast cancer of American women we could drop breast cancer by 90%.

FLAXSEED AND BREAST CANCER

A randomized double blind placebo controlled clinical trial of flaxseed in breast cancer patients finds flax appeared to have the potential to reduce tumor growth in just a few weeks and enhance survival.

Dr. Campbell, co-author of the China Study, found breast cancer was rare in rural China: 1 in 100,000, while in the west it's 1 in 8. China does not have a dairy infrastructure. Mushrooms consumption regularly is associated with a significantly decreased risk of breast cancer in both pre-and postmenopausal women. Frequent consumption of mushrooms can decrease the incidence of breast cancer by up to 60 to 70 percent! In one recent study, women who ate at least 10 grams of fresh mushrooms each day (equivalent to just one small mushroom) had a 64 percent decrease risk of breast cancer. Even more dramatic protection was gained by women who ate 10 grams of mushrooms and consumed green compounds from green tea daily--an 89 percent decrease in risk for premenopausal women and 82 percent for postmenopausal women. Why doesn't the whole world know this? (Raw mushrooms can be toxic lite cooking removes the risk and heat does not affect it's healing properties). One mechanism in which mushrooms reduce breast cancer risk by reducing the estrogen from stimulating breast tissue, aromatase is an enzyme that produces estrogen and is responsible for regulating estrogen levels in the body. Highest anti-aromatase activity: white button, white stuffing, cremini, Portobello, reishi, maitake.

Mushrooms also contain an angiogenesis inhibitor that further inhibits tumors and growth of abnormal cells, tumors, and cancers. Angiogenesis, means the growth of new blood vessels. Cancers, tumors, and fat secrete angiogenesis-promoting compounds that fuel their own growth; but mushrooms say no.

Vegetarian women have less breast cancer then women who eat the SAD one thing they have 2 or 3 bowel movements a day. Dr. Greger calls them super poppers. This helps rid the body of excess estrogen and cholesterol.

Prostate cancer is highest in African Americans 30 times greater than Japanese men and 120 times greater than Chinese men living in Shanghai. Maybe it's the diet.

FLAXSEED VS PROSTATE CANCER

Researchers studied 15 men who had just had their prostate biopsied and were scheduled to get a repeat biopsy in six months' time. They were put on a lowfat diet (less than 20% kcal) and flaxseed supplement (30g a day) and were provided with a supply to last throughout the six-month intervention period.

These were men with what's called PIN, which is like the prostate equivalent of ductal carcinoma tissue in the breast, an early stage of cancer. That's why they were getting repeat biopsy --to make sure it wasn't spreading. They found after 6 months a significant drop in PSA levels which is a biomarker of prostate cell growth and a significant decrease in cellular proliferation rate in fact in two of the men their PSA dropped so low they didn't have to go through with the second biopsy.

The allium family of vegetable, onions, garlic, leeks, shallots, chives and scallions: epidemiological studies have found that increased consumption of allium vegetables is associated with lower risk of cancer at all common sites.

For instance, onions: in a case-control multi country study, found the highest consumers of onions had less than half as many cancers compared to people who rarely consumed onions. Here are the specific stats:

- A 56 percent reduction in colon cancer

- A 73 percent reduction in ovarian cancer

- An 88 percent reduction in esophageal cancer

- A 71 percent reduction in prostate cancer

- A 50 percent reduction in stomach cancer

In this study the highest consumers were eating about a half a cup of chopped onions a day imagine the protective effects of eating adequate amounts of cruciferous greens, mushrooms, onions, and flaxseed almost daily.

Pomegranates inhibit breast cancer, prostate cancer, colon cancer and leukemia, and prevent vascular changes that promote tumor growth in lab animals.

Berries--strawberries, blueberries, raspberry, acai berries, goji berries, elderberries, and scientist discovered ellagic acid, found in many fruits and vegetables and berries, inhibited the formations of tumors. Berries also contained an assortment of anthocyanins with powerful anticancer effects.

Pancreatic cancer is often not detected until it's too late. A new test out of England where they check for certain markers in your urine is under way. Hopefully, it's perfected soon

All vegetables contain protective unique chemical composition but cruciferous vegetables have a unique chemical composition. When their cell walls are broken by blending or chopping a chemical reaction occurs that converts these sulfur-containing compound into isothiocyanates (ITC's) over 120 have been identified and the various ITCs have different mechanisms of action one ITC stops cancer cell growth or induce death in cancer cells such as those involved in breast and colon cancer.

PREVENTING AND TREATING BREAST CANCER

HOW TO PREVENT BREAST CANCER

The controversy over the cost and effectiveness of mammograms misses an important point: Breast cancer screening, by definition, does not prevent breast cancer. It can just pick up existing breast cancer. Based on autopsy studies, as many as 39 percent of women in their forties already have breast cancers growing within their bodies that may be simply too small to be detected by mammograms. That's why you can't just wait until diagnosis to start eating and living healthier. You should start now.

RISK FACTORS

The American Institute for Cancer Research (AICR) one of the world's leading authorities on diet and cancer. The ten recommendations for cancer prevention: Diets that revolve around whole plant foods-vegetables, whole grains, fruits and beans cut the risk of many cancers, and other diseases as well.

Researchers followed a group of about thirty thousand postmenopausal women with no history of breast cancer. They achieved just three of the ten AICR recommendations limiting alcohol, eating mostly plant foods, and maintaining a normal body weight these three simple health behaviors appeared to cut risk by 62%.

Pritikin researchers demonstrated that eating a plant based diet and walking every day can improve our cancer defenses within just two weeks. Researchers dripped the blood of women before and after fourteen days of healthy living onto breast cancer cells growing in petri dishes. The blood taken after they started eating healthier suppressed cancer growth significantly better and killed 20-30 percent more cancer cells than the blood taken from the same women just two weeks before. Researchers attributed this effect to a decrease in levels of a cancer-promoting growth hormone called IGF-1 likely due to the reduced intake of animal protein.

In 2010, the official World Health Organization body that assesses cancer risks upgraded its classification of alcohol to a definitive human breast carcinogen. In 2014 it clarified its position by stating that, regarding breast cancer, no amount of alcohol is safe.

Red wine a compound in red wine appears to suppress the activity of an enzyme called estrogen synthase, which breast tumors can use to create estrogen to fuel their own growth. This compound is found in the skin of the dark-purple grapes used to make red wine, which explains why white wine appears to provide no such benefit, since it's produced without the skin.

Melatonin The pineal gland setting in the middle of your brain has one function to produce melatonin. The pineal bland is inactive during the day but when it begins to get dark it activates and begins pumping melatonin into your bloodstream. Melatonin secretion may peak between 2:00 am and 5:00 am. The level of melatonin in your bloodstream is one of the ways your internal organs know what time it is. Melatonin is thought to play another role-surprising cancer. Researchers from Brigham and Women's Hospital in Boston thought that blind women can't see sunlight, their pineal glands never stop secreting melatonin into their bloodstreams. Yep the researchers found that blind women may have just half the odds of breast cancer as sighted women. Conversely, women who interrupt their melatonin production by working night shifts appear to be an increased risk for breast cancer. Even living on a particularly brightly lit street may affect the risk.

Melatonin production can be gauged by measuring the amount of melatonin excreted in our first pee in the morning and women with higher melatonin secretion have been found to have lower rates of breast cancer. Japanese researchers reported an association between higher vegetable intake and higher melatonin levels in urine. Harvard researchers in 2009 asked nearly a thousand women about their consumption of thirty-eight different foods or food groups and measured their morning melatonin levels. Meat consumption was the only food significantly associated with lower melatonin production, for reasons still unknown.

Exercise is considered a promising preventive measure against breast cancer it helps with weight control and tends to lower circulating estrogen levels. Five hours a week of vigorous aerobic exercise can lower estrogen and progesterone exposure by about 20 percent. Leisurely strolls don't appear to cut it. Walking at a moderate pace for an hour or more a day is associated with significantly lower breast cancer risk.

Heterocyclic Amines (HCAs) described by the National Cancer Institute as "chemicals formed when muscle meat, including beef, pork, fish, and poultry is cooked using high-temperature methods." These cooking methods include roasting, pan frying, grilling, and baking. People who eat meat that never goes above 212 degrees. Fahrenheit produce urine and feces that are significantly less DNA-damaging compared to those eating meat dry-cooked at higher temperatures. This means they have fewer mutagenic substances flowing through their bloodstreams and coming in contact with their colons.

These carcinogens are formed in a high-temperature chemical reaction between some of the components of muscle tissue. The longer meat is cooked, the more HCAs form. This process may explain why eating well-done meat is associated with increased risk of cancers of the breast, colon, esophagus, lung, pancreas, prostate, and stomach.

The situation creates what the Harvard Health s Letter called a meat preparation "paradox" Cooking meat thoroughly reduces the risk of contracting foodborne infections but cooking meat too thoroughly may increase the risk of foodborne carcinogens.

The carcinogens found in cooked meat are thought to explain why, as the Long Island Breast Cancer Study Project reported in 2007, women who eat more grilled, barbecued, or smoked meats over their lifetimes may have as much as 47 percent higher odds of breast cancer. And the Iowa Women's Health Study found that women who ate their bacon, beefsteak, and burgers "very well done" had nearly five times the odds of getting breast cancer compared with women who preferred these meats served rare or medium.

HCAs appear able both to initiate and to promote cancer growth. PhIP, one of the most abundant HCAs in cooked meat, was found to have potent estrogen like effects, fueling human breast-cancer cell growth almost as powerfully as pure estrogen, on which most human breast tumors thrive. (HCAs can also be found in fried eggs.)

Your body can rapidly rid itself of these toxins once exposure ceases. In fact. Urine levels of PhIP can drop to zero within twenty-four hours of refraining from eating meat.

Cholesterol Cancers appears to feed on cholesterol. LDL cholesterol stimulates the growth of breast cancer cells in a petri dish they just gobble up the so-called bad cholesterol. Tumors may suck up so much cholesterol that cholesterol levels tend to plummet as their cancer grows. This is not a good sign, as patient survival tends to be lowest when cholesterol uptake is highest.

The cancer is thought to be using the cholesterol to make estrogen or to shore up tumor membranes to help the cancer migrate and invade more tissue.

Data is mixed the largest study on cholesterol and cancer including more than a million participants found a 17 percent increased risk in women who had total cholesterol levels over 240 compared to women whose cholesterol was under 160. If lowering cholesterol may help what about cholesterol lowering statins.

Statins looked promising in petri-dish studies, but population studies comparing breast cancer rates among statin users and nonusers showed inconsistent results. Most consider 5 years to be long term statin use, but breast cancer can take decades to develop.

The first major study on the breast cancer risk of statin use for ten years or longer was published in 2013. It found that women who had been taking statins for a decade or more had twice the risk of both common types of infiltrating breast cancer: invasive ductal carcinoma and invasive lobular carcinoma. The cholesterol drugs doubled the risk. If confirmed, the public health implications of these findings are immense: Approximately one in four women in the united states over the age of forty-five may be taking these drugs.

The number one killer of women is heart disease, not breast cancer, so women still need to bring down their cholesterol. You can likely achieve this without drugs by eating a healthy enough plant-based diet. And certain plant foods may be particularly protective.

Bovine Leukemia Virus. The presence of bovine leukemia virus DNA in breast tissues was strongly associated with diagnosed and confirmed breast cancer. As many as 37% of breast cancer cases may be attributable to BLV exposure. As many as 37% of human breast cancer cases may be attributable to exposure to bovine leukemia virus.

What was the dairy industry response to that as many as 37% of breast cancer cases may be attributable to exposure to bovine leukemia virus, a cancer-causing cow virus, found in the milk of nearly every dairy herd in the United States.

The industry pointed out that some women without breast cancer harbored the virus, too. OK, the virus was also found in the tissues of 29% of women who did not have breast cancer-to which the researchers replied yet. It can take decades before a breast tumor can be picked up by mammography.

The cattle industry appeared more concerned about public confidence then public health.

BLV is a blood-borne virus. It's spread by unsanitary practices like using the same needle without sterilizing between cattle and other practices I don't care to discuss. BLV has been eradicated in 20 other countries.

PREVENTING AND TREATING BREAST CANCER WITH PLANT BASED DIET

Yale researchers found that premenopausal women who ate more than about six grams of soluble fiber a day (single cup of black beans) had 62% lower odds of breast cancer compared with women who consumed less than 4 grams a day. Fiber's benefits appeared even more effective for estrogen-receptor- negative breast tumors. Premenopausal women on a higher fiber diet had 85 percent lower odds of that type of breast cancer.

How did the researchers arrive at these figures? They asked them what they ate trying to tease out something distinctive about the eating habits of those women who developed the disease and those that did not. So maybe they were just eating less bacon.

A compilation of ten cohort studies on breast cancer and fiber intake came up with a 14 percent lower risk for breast cancer for every twenty grams of fiber intake per day. The relationship between more fiber and less breast cancer may not be a straight line. Breast cancer risk may not significantly fall until at least twenty-five grams of fiber a day is reached. The average American women appears to eat less than fifteen grams of fiber per day only about half the minimum daily recommendation.

An apple a day, The results of a study if eating an apple a day was associated with lower cancer risk compared with people who ate less than one apple a day. Daily apple eaters had a 24 percent lower odds of breast cancer, as well as significantly lower risk for ovarian cancer, laryngeal cancer, and colorectal cancer.

The cancer protection apples appear to offer is assumed to arise from their antioxidant properties which are concentrated in the peel.

Beyond protecting against the initial free-radical hit to your DNA, apple extract has been shown to suppress the growth of both estrogen-receptor-positive and-negative breast cancer cells in a petri dish. When researchers dripped extracts of peel and flesh from the same apples separately on cancer cells, the peel stopped cancer growth ten times more effectively.

Researchers found something in the peels that appears to reactivate a tumor-suppressor gene called maspin. Maspin is one of the tools your body appears to use to keep breast cancer at bay. Breast cancer cells find a way to turn off this gene, but apple peels appear to be able to turn it back on.

Cruciferous vegetables: Researchers fed a group of nonsmokers pan-fried meat. They then measured the levels of heterocyclic amines circulating in their bodies by sampling their urine. For two weeks, the study subjects added about three cups of broccoli and brussels sprouts to their daily diets and then ate the same meat meal. Through they consumed the same quantity of carcinogens, significantly less came out in their urine. Broccoli, brussels sprouts boost the liver's detox ability

The subjects stopped eating their vegetables and two weeks later, tried eating the meat meal again. Presuming their ability to detox carcinogens would by then reverted back to baseline. But instead, the subjects' liver function remained enhanced even weeks later.

A study of 50,000 African American women a population group who tends to regularly eat more greens found that those who ate two or more servings of vegetables a day had significantly decreased risk of a kind of breast cancer that's hard to treat, estrogen-and progesterone-receptor negative. Broccoli appeared especially protective among premenopausal women, but collard green consumption was associated with less breast cancer risk at all ages.

Flaxseeds Hippocrates wrote about using them to treat patients. Richest plant sources for essential omega-3 fatty acids. Flaxseeds have about 100 times more lignans than any other foods. Just like broccoli doesn't technically contain sulforaphane (only the precursors that turn into sulforapane when chewed) flaxseeds don't contain lignans, only lignin precursors which need to be activated by the good bacteria in your gut. Women with frequent urinary tract infections may be at a higher risk of breast cancer because every course of antibiotics you take can kill bacteria indiscriminately, it may stymie the ability of the good bacteria in your gut to take full advantage of the lignans in your diet.

Lignins are phytoestrogens that can dampen the effects of the body's own estrogen. In terms of breast cancer risk, eating about a daily tablespoon full of ground flaxseeds can extend a woman's menstrual cycle by about a day. This means she'll have fewer periods over the course of a life time. And, therefore, presumably less estrogen exposure and reduced breast cancer risk.

Lignin intake is associated with significantly reduced breast cancer risk in postmenopausal women. This effect is presumed to be due to lignans' further estrogen-dampening effects. But since lignans are found in healthy foods like berries whole grains, and dark, leafy greens, could they just be an indicator of a healthy diet.

The strongest evidence to date that there really is something special about this class of phytonutrients comes from interventional trials, starting with a 2010 study funded by the National Cancer Institute. Researchers took about forty-five women at high risk of breast cancer-meaning they had suspicious breast biopsies or had previously suffered from breast cancer-and gave they the equivalent of about two teaspoons of ground flaxseeds every day. Needle biopsies of breast tissue were taken before and after the yearlong study. The results: On average the women had fewer precancerous changes in their breasts after the year of flax lignans than before they started. Eighty percent (thirty-six of forty-five) had a drop in their levels of Ki-67, a biomarker (indicator) of increased cell proliferation. This finding suggests that sprinkling a few spoonfuls of ground flaxseeds on your oatmeal or whatever you're eating throughout the day may reduce the risk of breast cancer.

Breast cancer survivors who have higher levels of lignans in their bloodstreams and diets appear to survive significantly longer. This outcome may be due to the fact that women who eat flaxseeds may also see a rise in the levels of endostatin in their breasts. Endostatin is a protein produced by your body to help starve tumors of their blood supply.

Evidence appeared so compelling that scientists performed a randomized, double-blind, placebo-controlled clinical trial of flaxseeds for breast cancer patients—one of the few times a food has ever been so rigorously put to the test. Researchers located women with breast cancer scheduled for surgery and divided them randomly into two groups: Every day, group one ate a muffin containing flaxseed, while group two ate a muffin that looked and tasted the same, but had no flaxseed,in it. Biopsises of the tumors in the flax and no-flax groups were taken at the beginning of the study and then compared with the pathology of the tumor removed during surgery about five weeks later.

Compared with the women who ate the placebo muffins, women consuming the muffins with flaxseed, on average, witnessed their tumor-cell proliferation decreased, cancer-cell death rates increase, and their c-erB2 scores go down. C-erB2 is a marker of cancer aggressiveness; the higher your score, the higher the potential for breast cancer to metastasize and spread throughout the body. In other words, the flaxseeds appeared to make the subjects' cancer less aggressive. The researchers concluded, "Dietary flaxseed has the potential to reduce tumor growth in patients with breast cancer. Flaxseed, may be a potential dietary alternative or adjunct to currently used breast cancer drugs.

Breast Cancer Stem Cells What if you're already fighting breast cancer or are in remission? Scientists have been developing a new theory of cancer biology over the past decade based on the role of stem cells. Stem cells are foundational material from which all other cells with specialized functions are generated. Stem cells are a critical component of the body's repair system, including regrowing skin, bone, and muscle. Breast tissue naturally has many stem cells in reserve, which are used during pregnancy to create new milk glands. As miraculous as stem cells are, their immortality can also work against us. Instead of rebuilding organs, if they turn cancerous, they can build tumors.

Cancerous stem cells may be why breast cancer can return, even up to twenty-five years after being fought off successfully the first time. When people are told that they are cancer-free, it may mean their tumors are gone, but if their stem cells are cancerous, the tumors still might reappear many years later. Sadly, someone who has been cancer-free for ten years might consider herself cured but actually may just be in remission. Cancerous stem cells may be just waiting to reignite.

The current sophisticated chemo drugs and radiation regimens is based on animal models. Success of a given treatment is often measured by its ability to shrink tumors In rodents—rats only live for about two or three years in any case. Doctors may be shrinking tumors, but mutated stem cells may still be lurking, able to slowly rebuild new tumors over the ensuing years.

We need to do is attack the root of cancer not just at reducing tumor bulk but at targeting what has been called the "beating heart of the tumor" cancer stem cells.

Broccoli may help or more specific sulforaphane, adietary component of cruciferous vegetables like broccoli, has been shown to suppress the ability of breast cancer stem cells to form tumors. This means if you're currently in remission, eating lots of broccoli could theoretically help keep your cancer from returning. (Theoretically because those results were from a petri dish.)

Researchers at John Hopkins if sulforaphane would be absorbed in your blood stream when you eat broccoli. The researchers asked women scheduled for breast reduction surgery to drink broccoli-sprout juice an hour before their procedure. After dissecting their breast tissue post surgery, the researchers found evidence of significant sulforaphane buildup. They now know that the cancer fighting nutrients in broccoli do find their way to right place when we swallow them.

To reach the concentration of sulforaphane in the breast found to suppress breast caner stem cells, you would have to eat at least a quarter cup of broccoli sprouts a day. They are cheap and you can grow them at home.

There have been no randomized clinical trials to see if breast cancer survivors who eat broccoli live longer than those who don't but you have no downside and only positive side effects.

Soy and Breast Cancer Soybeans naturally contain another class of phytoestrogens called isoflavones. Phytoestrogens dock into the same receptors as your own estrogen but have a weaker effect, so they can act to block the effects of your more powerful animal estrogen.

There are two types of estrogen receptors in the body, alpha and beta. Your own estrogen prefers alpha receptors, while plant estrogens have an affinity for the beta receptors. The effects of soy phytoestrogens on different tissues therefore depend on the ratio of alpha to beta receptors.

Estrogen has positive effects in some tissues and potentially negative effects in others. For example, high levels of estrogen can be good for the bones but can increase the likelihood of developing breast cancer. Ideally, you'd like what's called a selective estrogen receptor modulator in your body that would have progestogenic effects in some tissues and antiestrogenic effects in others.

That's what soy phytoestrogens appear to be. Soy seems to lower breast cancer risk, and antiestrogenic effect, but can also help reduce menopausal hot-flash symptoms, a progestogenic effect. So, by eating soy, you may be able to enjoy the best of both worlds.

Soy for women with breast cancer. There have been five studies on breast cancer survivors and soy consumption. Researchers have found that women diagnosed with breast cancer who ate the most soy lived significantly longer and had significantly lower risk of breast cancer recurrence than those who ate less. The quantity of phytoestrogens found in just a single cup of soy milk may reduce the risk of breast cancer returning by 25 percent. The improvement in survival for those eating more soy foods was found both in women whose tumors were responsive to estrogen (estrogen-receptor positive breast cancer). This also held true for both young women and older women. In one study, 90 percent of the breast cancer patients who ate the most soy phytoestrogens after diagnosis were still alive five years later, while half of those who ate little to no soy were dead.

One way soy may decrease cancer risk and improve survival is by helping to reactivate BRCA genes. BRCA1 and BRAC2 are so-called caretaker genes, cancer-suppressing genes responsible for DNA repair. Mutations in this gene can cause a rare form of hereditary breast cancer. As has been well publicized, Angelina Jolie decided to undergo a preventive double mastectomy. A National Breast Cancer Coalition survey found that the majority of women believe that most breast cancers occur among women with a family history or a genetic predisposition to the disease. The reality is that as few as 2.5 percent of breast cancer cases are attributable to breast cancer running in the family.

The vast majority of breast cancer patients have fully functional BRAC genes, meaning that their DNA-repair mechanisms are intact, how did their breast cancer form, grow and spread? Breast Tumors appear able to suppress the expression of the gene through a process called methylation. While the gene itself is operational, the cancer has effectively turned it off or at least turned down its expression, potentially aiding the metastatic spread of a tumor.

The isoflavones in soy appear to help turn BRCA protection back on, removing the methyl straitjacket the tumor tried to place on it. The dose used by researchers in vitro to achieve this results was the equivalent to eating about a cup of soybeans.

Soy may help with variations of other breast cancer susceptibility genes known as MDM2. And CYP1B1. Women at increased genetic risk of breast cancer may benefit from high soy intake.

No matter which genes you inherit, changes in your diet may be able to affect DNA expression at a genetic level, potentially boosting your ability to fight disease.

Why do Women is Asia have less breast cancer. Asian women are up to 5 times less likely to develop breast cancer than North American women one possibility is their intake of green tea a common staple in many Asian diets. Green tea has been associated with about a 30 percent reduction in breast cancer risk. Another strong possibility is a relatively high intake of soy, which, is consumed consistently during childhood, may cut the risk of breast cancer later in life by half. If women consume soy primarily as an adult, though, their risk reduction may only be closer to 25 percent. Asian populations also eat more mushrooms. Researchers decided to investigate if there was a link between mushroom intake and breast cancer. They compared the mushroom consumption of one thousand breast cancer patients to one thousand healthy subjects of similar age, weight, and smoking and exercise status. The women whose mushroom consumption averaged just about one-half a mushroom or more per day had 64 percent lower odds of breast cancer compared with women who didn't eat mushrooms at all. Eating mushrooms and sipping at least half a tea bag's worth of green tea each day was associated with nearly 90 percent lower breast cancer odds.

In medicine, a cancer diagnosis is considered a "teachable moment" when doctors can motivate a patient to improve his or her lifestyle. By then, though, it may already be too late.

NEW BLOOD TEST FOR CANCER

The ONCOblot Test is a highly sensitive blood test for cancer. It confirms the presence of cancer as well as the tissue of origin through the detection of EMOX2 proteins. ENOX2 proteins are detected 4-10 years in advance of clinical symptoms.

The ENOX2 protein species in the blood is unique to malignant cells and absent from non-cancer cells. These proteins can be detected in early development. The ONCOblot test identifies the ENOX2 markers and the direct visualization of a marker presence significantly reduces false positives.

The ONCOblot test reveals the tissue of origin of the ENOX2 protein. The ONCOblot database contains the following 25+cancers:

Bladder	Leukemia	Pancreatic
Breast	Non-Small cell	Prostate
Cervical	Lung Small cell	Sarcoma
Endometrial	Lymphoma	Squamous Cell
Esophageal	Melanoma	Follicular Thyroid
Gastric	Mesothelloma	Papillary Thyroid
Hepatocelluar	Myelom	Testicular Germ Cell
Kidney	Ovarian	Uterine
Colorectal		

HIGH BLOOD PRESSURE

The most comprehensive and systematic analysis of the causes of death ever undertaken was published recently in Lancet, one of the world's leading medical journals. Funded by the Bill and Melinda Gates Foundation, the Global Burden of Disease Study involved nearly five hundred researchers from more than three hundred institutions in fifty countries and examined nearly one hundred thousand data sources. The results allow us to answer such questions as "How many lives could we save if people around the world cut back on soda?" The best answer 299,521. So soft drinks and their empty calories don't just fail to promote health- they actually seem to promote death. But apparently, soda isn't nearly as deadly as bacon, bologna, ham, and hot dogs. Processed meat is blamed for the deaths of more than eight hundred thousand people every year. Worldwide, that's four times more people than who die from illicit drug use.

The study also noted which foods, if added to the diet, might save lives. Eating more whole grains could potentially save 1.7 million lives a year. More vegetables? 1.8 million lives. How about nuts and seeds? 2.5 million lives. The researchers didn't look at beans, but of the foods they considered, which does the world need most? Fruit. Worldwide, if humanity ate more fruit, we might save 4.9 million lives. That's nearly 5 million lives hanging in the balance, and their salvation isn't medication or a new vaccine- it may be just more fruit.

The number-one risk factor for death in the world they identified is high blood pressure. Also known as hypertension, high blood pressure lays waste to nine million people worldwide every year. It kills so many people because it contributes to deaths from a variety of causes, including aneurysms, heart attack, heart failure, kidney failure, and stroke.

In the United States, nearly seventy-eight million people have high blood pressure- that's about one in three Americans and 80% of type 2 diabetes have high blood pressure.

In the 1920s, researchers measured the blood pressure of a thousand native Kenyans who ate a low-sodium diet centered around whole plant foods—whole grains, fruits, and dark, leafy greens, and other vegetables. Up until age forty, the blood pressure of the rural Africans was similar to that of Europeans and Americans, about 125/80. However, as Westerners aged, their blood pressure began to surge past the Kenyans. By age sixty, the average Westerner was hypertensive, with blood pressure exceeding 140/90. What about the Kenyans? By age sixty, their average blood pressure had actually improved to an average of about 110/70.

The 140/90 threshold for hypertension is considered an arbitrary cutoff. Just like having too much cholesterol or body fat, there are benefits to having a blood pressure that is even lower than the normal range. So even people who start out with so-called normal blood pressure of 120/80 appear to benefit from going down to 110/70. But it is possible to do that? Look at the Kenyans--not only is it possible, it appears typical for people who live healthy, plant-based lifestyles.

Over a two-year period, 1,800 patients were admitted into a rural Kenyan hospital. How many cases of high blood pressure did they find? ZERO. There also wasn't a single case found of America's number-one killer, atherosclerosis.

The two most prominent dietary risks for death and disability in the world may be not eating enough fruit and eating too much salt. Nearly five million people appear to die every year as a result of not eating enough fruit, while eating too much salt.

The American Heart Association recommends everyone consume less than 1,500 mg of sodium daily -that's about three-quarters of a teaspoon of salt. The average American adult consumes more than double that amount about 3,500 mg daily. Reducing sodium consumption by just 15 percent worldwide could save millions of lives every year.

If we could cut our salt intake by about a half teaspoon a day, which is achievable by avoiding salty foods and not adding salt to our food, we might prevent 22 percent of stroke deaths and 16 percent of fatal heart attacks. That's potentially more lives saved than if we were able to successfully treat people with blood pressure pills. Reducing salt is an easy at-home intervention that may be more powerful than filling a prescription from the pharmacy. Up to 92,000 Americans lives could be saved each year simply by eating less salt.

Before the invention of blood pressure lowering drugs people literally would die from out of control blood pressure (known as malignant hypertension) a condition from which go blind from bleeding into your eyes, your kidneys shut down, and your heart eventually fails.

Dr. Walter Kempner, a Prussian who fled Nazi Germany and set up practice at Duke University, with his rice and fruit diet to treat malignant hypertension which was a death sentence, with a life expectance of about six months. Nevertheless, he was able to reverse the course of disease with diet in more than 70 percent of cases. Without drugs, he brought patients with blood pressure like 240/150 down to 105/80 with dietary changes alone.

Salty meals can significantly impair artery function. Salt itself can injure our arteries independent of its impact on blood pressure. It turns out that sodium intake appears to suppress the activity of a key antioxidant enzyme in the body called superoxide dismutase, which has the ability to detoxify a million free radicals per second. With the action of this workhorse of an enzyme stifled by sodium, artery-crippling levels of oxidative stress can build up.

The salt industry isn't thrilled about the idea of our cutting back on salt. When the American Heart Association quoted the chair of the U.S. Dietary Guidelines Advisory Committee as saying that Americans should reduce their sodium intake., the Salt Institute, a salt industry trade organization, accused her of having an "unhealthy prejudice" against salt, arguing that she had "pre-judged the salt issue". This is like the tobacco industry complaining that people at the American Lung Association are biased against smoking. Of course, the Salt Institute wasn't the only aggrieved party. Cheese, it turns out, ranks as a leading contributor of sodium in the American diet, and the National Dairy Council stood shoulder-to-shoulder with Big Salt in its condemnation of the Dietary Guidelines Advisory Committee recommendations.

The salt industry has its own PR and lobbying firms to play tobacco industry-style tactics to downplay the dangers of its product. But the real villains are the processed food industry. The trillion-dollar processed food industry uses dirt-cheap added salt and sugar to sell us their junk. That's why it's not easy avoiding sodium on the typical American diet, since three-quarters of salt come from processed foods rather than a saltshaker. By hooking you on hyper sweet and hyper salty foods, your taste buds get so dampened that natural foods can taste like cardboard.

But there are two other major reasons the food industry adds salt to foods. If you add salt to meat, it draws in water. This way, a company can increase the weight of its product by nearly 20 percent. Since meat is sold by the pound, that's 20 percent more profits for very little added cost. Second, as everyone knows, eating salt makes us thirsty. There's a reason bars put out free baskets of salted nuts and pretzels, and it's the same reason soda conglomerates like Pepsi and Frito-Lay are part of the same corporation.

The poultry industry commonly injects chicken carcasses with salt water to artificially inflate their weight, yet they can still be labelled "100 percent natural." Consumer Reports found that some supermarket chickens were pumped so full of salt that they registered a whopping 840 mg of sodium per serving-which could mean more than a full day's worth of sodium in just one chicken breast.

The number one source of sodium for American kids and teens is pizza. A single slice of Pizza Hut pepperoni pizza can contain half your recommended sodium intake limit for the entire day. For adults over fifty, it's bread, but between the ages of twenty and fifty, the greatest contributor of sodium to the diet is chicken-not the canned soups, pretzels, or potato chips one might expect.

How can you overcome your craving for salt, sugar, and fat? Just give it a few weeks, and your taste buds will start to change. When researchers put people on a low- salt diet, over time, the research subjects increasingly enjoyed the taste of salt-free soup and became turned off by the salt-heavy soup they had previously craved.

The same may be true for sugar and fat. It's likely that humans actually taste fat, just like they taste sweet, sour, and salty flavors. People placed on low fat diets start preferring low-fat foods over fatty options. Pritikin said you can retrain your palate in about 30 days. Even non-fast food restaurants tend to pile on the salt and avoid processed foods.

Whole Grains: On average, high blood pressure medications reduce the risk of heart attack by 15 percent and the risk of stroke by 25 percent. But in a randomized, controlled trial, three portions of whole grains a day were able to help people achieve this blood-pressure-lowering benefit too. The study revealed that a diet rich in whole grains yields the same benefits without the adverse side effects commonly associated with antihypertensive drugs, such as electrolyte disturbances in those taking diuretics (also known as water pills), increased breast cancer risk for those taking calcium-channel blockers (like Norvasc or Cardizem), lethargy and impotence for those on beta blockers (like Lopressor and Corgard), sudden, potentially life -threatening swelling for those taking ACE inhibitors (like Vasotec and Altace), and an increased risk of serious fall injuries for apparently any class of these blood pressure drugs.

Whole grains do have side effects, though. Good ones! Whole-grain intake is associated with lower risks of type 2 diabetes, coronary heart disease, weight gain, and colon cancer. Take note of the whole, however. While whole grains such as oats, whole wheat, and brown rice, have been shown to reduce your risk of developing chronic disease, refined grains may actually increase your risk. Harvard researchers, for example, found that while regular consumption of brown rice was associated with a lower risk of type 2 diabetes, consuming white rice was associated with higher risk. Daily servings of white rice were associated with a 17 percent greater risk of diabetes, whereas replacing a serving a day of white rice with brown rice might lead to a 16 percent drop in risk. And it looks like replacing white rice with oats and barley may be an even more powerful step, associated with a 36 percent drop in diabetes risk.

High blood pressure patients commonly end up on three different antihypertensive drugs at a time, yet only about half tend to stick to even the first-line drugs. (This is due in part to all their side effects which can include erectile dysfunction, fatigue, and leg cramps.) At the end of all of this the drugs still haven't gotten to the root cause of the problem. The cause of high blood pressure isn't medication deficiency. The underlying cause is what you eat and how you live.

The ideal blood pressure, defined as the level at which lowering it further yields no additional benefit, is probably around 110/70. Can you really get it that low without medication? This is the average blood pressure of men more than sixty years old in rural Africa on no treatment other than their traditional, plant-based diets and lifestyles. In rural China, we find similar results: 110/70 throughout life without any increase with age. The only group in the Western world able to achieve routinely these blood pressure readings are vegetarians.

Additional hypertension protection; flaxseeds, hibiscus tea, and nitrate-rich vegetables. Ground flaxseeds alone "induced one of the most potent blood-pressure lowering effects ever achieved by a dietary intervention. Eating just a few tablespoons a day appears to be two to three times more powerful than adopting an aerobic endurance exercise program but you should do both."

Pritikin in his lost lectures discusses a study the doctor reduced the test group's fat intake by 20 percent-- no sodium reduction no weight loss-- only change fat intake blood pressure dropped 10 percent.

BUG ASSAULT THE ONLY TIME I USE SALT

The day my Bug Assault gun arrived I changed into a camouflage T-shirt and hat. I ordered the camouflage model because flies have about 100 eyes. The gun is air powered and shoots a small charge of salt. I opened the kitchen door and cut a chilled piece of watermelon sat down at my kitchen table with my Bug Assault Gun on my lap. Then my girlfriend came over she's an attorney. Gary,did you know your door is wide open? Your letting flies in! "Let them come" I'm hunting flies raised my Bug Assault gun. Isn't the watermelon like hunting on a baited field yes but I don't think the law applies to flies. I'm going for a run you want to join me? nope I'm hunting flies raise my Bug assault gun again. How long are you going to be hunting? Until I get my limit. What's the limit I don't know. O.K. well we can discuss your hunt over dinner. Great, I'll cook, love you.

DEPRESSION

One hundred and fifty million people worldwide suffer from depression. Exercise vs. drugs for depression Men and women over 50 with major depression were randomized to either do an aerobic exercise program for four months, or take an antidepressant drug called Zoloft. They started out with Hamilton Depression scores up around 18 anything over seven is considered depressed. But within four months, the drug group came down too normal, which is exactly what the drugs are supposed to do. The exercise-only group, no drugs? Same powerful effect. Researchers did the largest study ever with three groups one group exercised together, one group exercised on their own and the drug group. And they all worked about just as well in terms of forcing the depression into remission.

So exercise is comparable to antidepressant medication in the treatment of patients with major depressive disorder.

Putting all the best studies together, the evidence indicates that exercise, at least, has a moderate antidepressant effect, and at best, exercise has a large effect on reductions in depression symptoms and could be categorized as a very useful and powerful intervention. Unfortunately, while studies support the use of exercise as a treatment for depression, exercise is rarely prescribed as a treatment for this common and debilitating problem. (Agarwal et al., 2015)

Depression may be a symptom of other health issues gluten sensitivity, fibromyalgia, deficiency of the amino acid tryptophan, B-12 deficiency, low testosterone, mercury (mostly from fish) artificial sweetener aspartame. Depression may be a risk factor for Alzheimer's disease and heart disease.

PLANT BASED DIETS FOR IMPROVED MOOD AND PRODUCTIVITY

Overweight men and women were randomized into a low-carb, high-fat diet, or high-carb, low fat diet for a year. By the end of the year who had less depression, anxiety, anger, and hostility, feelings of dejection, tension, fatigue, better vigor, less confusion, or mood disturbances? The low fat group and this is consistent with results from epidemiological studies showing that diets high in carbohydrate and low in fat and protein are associated with lower levels of anxiety and depression, and have beneficial effects on psychological wellbeing.

But the overall amount of fat in their diet didn't significantly change in this study, though. But the type of fat did. Their arachidonic acid intake fell to Zero.

Arachidonic acid is an inflammatory omega-6 fatty acid that can adversely impact mental health via a cascade of neuroinflammation. It may inflame your brain. High blood levels in the bloodstream have been associated with a greater likelihood of suicide risk, for example, and major depressive episodes. How can we stay away from the stuff?

Americans are exposed to arachidonic acid primarily through chicken and eggs. But when we remove chicken and eggs, and other meat, we can eliminate preformed arachidonic acid from our diet.

Dr. Neal Barnard set up study with a major insurance corporation Overweight or diabetic employees received either weekly group instruction on a whole food plant-based diet or no diet instruction for five months. There was no portion size restriction, no calorie counting, no carb counting. No change in exercise. No meals were provided, but the company cafeteria did start offering daily options such as lentil soup, minestrone, and bean burritos.

No meat, eggs, dairy, oil, or junk, yet they reported greater diet satisfaction compared with the control group participants who had no diet restrictions. How did they do? More participants in the plant-based intervention group reported improved digestion, increased energy, and better sleep than usual at week 22 compared with the control group. They also reported a significant increase in physical functioning, general health, vitality, and mental health.:

There were also significant improvements in work productivity, thought to be due, in large part, to their improvements in health. So, what this study demonstrated was that a cholesterol-free diet is acceptable, not only in research settings, but in a typical corporate environment, improving quality of life and productivity at little cost.

Then ten corporate sites across the country same kind of setup as before. Can it improve depression, anxiety, and productivity? Yes, significant improvements in depression, anxiety, fatigue, emotional well-being Life style interventions have an increasingly apparent role in physical and mental health, and among the most effective of these is a plant based diets.

According to the latest from the CDC, the rates of all of our top ten killers have fallen or stabilized except for one: suicide.

Accumulating evidence indicates that oxidative free radicals may play important roles in the development of various neuropsychiatric disorders, including major depression.

Lycopene, the red pigment predominantly found in tomatoes, but also present in watermelon, pink grapefruit, guava, and papaya, is the most powerful antioxidant amongst the carotenoid family. In a test tube, it's about 100 times more effective as quenching free radicals than vitamin E, for example.

And in a study of about a thousand older men and women, those who ate the most tomato products had about half the odds of depression. The researcher conclude that a tomato-rich diet may have a beneficial effect on the prevention of depressive symptoms.

Higher consumption of fruits and vegetables has been found to lead to a lower risk of developing depression, but if it's the antioxidants, can't we just take an antioxidant pill? Only food sources of antioxidants were protectively associated with depression. Not antioxidants from dietary supplements. Although plant foods and food-derived phytochemicals have been associated with health benefits, antioxidants from dietary supplements appear to be less beneficial, and may, in fact, be detrimental to health. This may indicate that the form and delivery of the antioxidants are important. Alternatively, the observed associations may be due not to antioxidants, but rather to other dietary factors, such as folate, which also occur in fruits and vegetables, and plant-rich diets.

In a study of thousands of middle-aged office workers, eating lots of processed food was found to be a risk factor for a least mild to moderate depression five years later, whereas a whole food pattern was found to be protective. Yes, it could be because of the high content of antioxidants in fruits and vegetables but could also be the folate in greens and beans, as some studies have suggested an increased risk of depression in folks who may not have been getting enough.

Low folate levels in the blood are associated with depression, the researchers didn't know if the low folate led to depression, or the depression led to low folate. Maybe when you have the blues, you don't want to eat the greens.

A number of cohort studies were published following people over time, and low dietary intake of folate may indeed be a risk factor for severe depression-as much as threefold higher risk. Note this is dietary folate intake, not folic acid supplements, so they were actually eating healthy foods. If you give people folic acid pills they don't seem to work. This may be because folate is found in dark green leafy vegetables like spinach, whereas folic acid is the oxidized synthetic compound used in food fortification and dietary supplements because it's more shelf-stable, but it may have different effects on the body. (Harnly et al., 2006)

ANTI-INFLAMMATORY DIET FOR TREATMENT OF DEPRESSION

Can an anti-inflammatory diet help prevent depression? About 45,000 women without depression were followed, along with their diets, for about a dozen years to see who became depressed, and it was those who ate a more inflammatory dietary pattern, characterized by more soda, refined grains and meat, suggesting that chronic inflammation may underlie the association between diet and depression. Normally, we think of omega-3's as anti-inflammatory, but they found fish on our mental well-to be pro-inflammatory, associated with increased c-reactive protein levels consistent with recent findings that omega-3's do not seem to help with either depression or inflammation. The most anti-inflammatory diet is a plant-based diet, which can cut C-reactive protein levels by 30% within two weeks, perhaps because of the anti-inflammatory properties of antioxidants. Now analyses of the published data and the unpublished data that were hidden by the drug companies reveals that most (if not all) of the benefits of antidepressants are due to the placebo effect.

And what's even worse, Freedom of Information Act documents show the FDA knew about it, but made an explicit decision to keep this information from the public and from prescribing physicians. How can this happen?

The pharmaceutical industry is considered the most profitable and politically influential industry and mental illness can be thought of as the drug industry's golden goose: incurable, common, long term, and involving multiple medications, Antidepressant medications are prescribed to 8.7% of the U.S. population.

There is strong therapeutic response to antidepressant medication: it's just that the response to placebo is almost as strong. Indeed, antidepressants offer substantial benefits to millions of people suffering from depression. To cast them as ineffective is inaccurate. Just because they may not work better than fake pills did not mean they don't work. It's like homeopathy. Just because it doesn't work better than the sugar pills that they are doesn't mean that homeopathy doesn't work, because the placebo effect is real and is powerful.

A psychiatrist funded by the Prozac company defends the drugs. A key issue is disregarded by the naysaying critics. If the patient is benefiting from antidepressant treatment, does it matter whether this is being achieved via drug or placebo effects?

Speaking of Prozac A double blind, randomized trial: Saffron versus Prozac. For 6 weeks 40 outpatients diagnosed with clinical depression got capsules containing the spice saffron-or, identical looking capsules containing Prozac. Within just one week a significant drop in depression symptoms that got better and better throughout the 6 weeks. Both were equally effective. 20% of the Prozac group suffered sexual dysfunction whereas no one did in the saffron group.

First, I think they have some oath first do no harm antidepressants caused sexual dysfunction, long-term weight gain, insomnia, nausea, and diarrhea. About one in five show withdrawal symptoms when they try to quit. More tragically, they may make people more likely to become depressed in the future. More likely to become depressed again after treatment by antidepressants than by treatment of other means including placebo.

Maybe doctors should give them actual sugar pills

If different treatments are equally effective, then shouldn't the choice be based on risk and harm? Antidepressant drugs may be the riskiest and most harmful, if they are to be used at all it should be as a last resort, when depression is extremely severe and all other treatment alternatives have been tried and failed.

Antidepressants may not work better than placebo for mild and moderate depression, but for very severe depression, the drugs do beat out sugar pills. That's just a small fraction of the people taking these drugs. That means that the vast majority of depressed patients maybe nine out of ten are being prescribed medications that have negligible benefits to them.

Too many doctors just quickly decide upon a depression diagnosis without necessarily listening to what the patient has to say, and they end up putting them on antidepressants without considering alternatives. And fortunately, there are effective alternatives. Physical exercise, for example, can have lasting effects, and if that turns out to also be the placebo effect, it is at least a placebo with an enviable list of side effects. (Kirsch, 2014)

PROBIOTICS AND MENTAL HEALTH

Over a century ago there were reports of successfully treating psychiatric illnesses like depression with a dietary regimen that included probiotics and put on a vegetarian diet and the people did feel better less depression, anger and hostility. better psychologically.

The field of inquiry remained dormant for about a hundred years, but a new discipline has recently emerged known as enteric-meaning intestinal-neuroscience. Our enteric nervous system, the collection of nerves in our gut has been referred to as our "second brain." We've got as many nerves in our gut as in our spinal cord. The size and complexity of our gut brain is not surprising when considering the challenges posed by the interface...with our largest body surface. We have a hundred times more contact with the outside world through our gut than through our skin. And we also have 100 trillion bacteria down there.

We know from an innovative study that looked at feces scraped from used toilet paper in undergrads during exam week, that our mental state can affect our gut, but can our gut affect our mental state?

This is the study that rocked the scientific establishment. An assessment of the psychotropic properties of probiotics. One month of probiotics was found to significantly decrease symptoms of anxiety, depression, anger and hostility. A variety of mechanisms have been proposed for how intestinal bacteria may be communicating with our brain.

Until that study was published, the idea that probiotic bacteria administered to the intestine could influence the brain seemed almost surreal. Likely, organisms already inside us carry out some degree of influence on our mental well-being. So might people suffering from certain forms of mental health problems benefit from a fecal transplant from someone with a more happy go luck bacteria? They don't know, but this ability of probiotics to affect brain processes is an exciting recent development in probiotic research.

William Styron author of Sophie's Choice, and other acclaimed works. In the summer of 1985, when he turned 60, he suddenly found that alcohol no longer agreed with him. But giving it up brought on mood disorders for which he had to be medicated. These drugs in turn produced destructive side effects and he was dragged into a deep, prolonged suicidal depression that did not lift until he was hospitalized from December through early February 1986.

He recovered and wrote a harrowing account of his experience which began as a lecture and became the bestselling book "Darkness Visible: A Memoir of Madness" (1990)

Depression continued to stalk him, and he was hospitalized several more times. In "Darkness Visible," he concluded, referring to Dante: "For those who have dwelt in depression's dark wood, and known its inexplicable agony, their return from the abyss is not unlike the ascent of the poet, trudging upward and upward out of hell's black depths and at last emerging into what he saw as "the shining world." There, whoever has been restored to health has almost always been restored to the capacity for serenity and joy, and this may be indemnity enough for having endured the despair beyond despair.

The pain of severe depression is quite unimaginable to those who have not suffered it and it kills in many instances because it's anguish can no longer be Bourne.

William Styron: "In Clinical depression, "he said "the psychological element merges into a chemical imbalance. Brain chemistry goes haywire, and when that happens it is catastrophic, an explosion in the mind, like the space shuttle challenger going off in midair. Stress and anxiety have an effect on your brain's neurotransmitters, removing from your consciousness any ability to receive impulses of pleasure. A palpable shroud of melancholy descends on you and becomes a pain as severe as a crushed knee. You cannot bear living any longer. The act of daily living, the whole diurnal process, becomes such a struggle you want to get out of it.

I shall never learn what caused my depression, it will likely forever prove to be an impossibility, when I arrived at the hospital via an air ambulance my brain tempest appeared to me so profound my standard joke I would rather have a bottle in front of me then a frontal lobotomy the later seemed almost acceptable. The self-medicating with Klonopin and Johnny Walker Red to keep the abyss at bay was not working only accelerating the dementia. A genetic component was present in my family, an unresolved loss existed in my past, stress of work. The guilt for everything I had ever done my sins seemed unpardonable. The pathways are too numerous for one single cause.

The hospital was my sanctuary I gradually but steadily got better fantasies of self-destruction all but disappeared within a few days. This was a place where peace could return to my mind.

Drugs and psychotherapy, in my case did little to bring me out of such despair. The support of family, friends and my girlfriend Lisa was far greater help. I can't imagine anything more horrible than suffering through depression alone.

By far the great majority of the people who go through even the severest depression survive it, and live ever afterward at least as happily as their unaffiliated counterparts. Save for the awfulness of certain memories it leaves, acute depression inflicts few permanent wounds. Those who are devastated once are often struck again; as many as half, depression has a habit of recurrence. But most victims live through even these relapses, often coping better because they have become psychologically tuned by past experience to deal with the ogre.

The endangered one can nearly always be saved. Most people in the grip of depression for whatever reason, are in a state of unrealistic hopelessness, exasperated ills and fatal threats and they bear no resemblance to actuality. It may require on the part of friends, lovers, family, admirers, an almost religious devotion to persuade the sufferers of life's worth, which is so often in conflict with a sense of their own worthlessness, but such devotion has prevented countless suicides.

Dr. Fuhrman, from his lecture "Disease Specific Nutritional Solutions" suggest Depression is largely nutritional and environmental. He recommends eating a whole food plant based diet, using lite therapy between 7 and 8 am to shut off the body's melatonin production and consolidate it, sleep in a dark room without electronics because they emit blue light. The bright light therapy also triggers serotonin and add an EPA supplement. Last but not least exercise.

PREVENTING ALZHEIMER'S

Alzheimer's is now the 6th leading cause of death in America. Based on autopsies, of thousands one can see what appears to be the first silent stages starting even in our 20s in about 10% of the population, and about 50% by age 50. These plaques and tangles the presence of these may constitute a true threat. The first stage of the disease has an extraordinarily long duration. Most people don't get diagnosed with Alzheimer's until their 70s. They now understand that neurodegenerative brain changes begin by middle age and so does cognitive decline. We start losing brain function in our 40s.

First people are diagnosed with what's called MCI, mild cognitive impairment. That's when cognitive decline become clinically apparent. A few years later Alzheimer's may be diagnosed, which then results in death. They did not know what was happening before mild cognitive impairment was diagnosed. There appears to be a slow decline in brain function and the buildup of plaques and tangles in the brain, for decades before Alzheimer's is diagnosed. This finding has profound implications for the prevention of dementia, we have to start early, before marked brain loss has occurred.

The good news is that brain disease is not inevitable, even after age 100. The oldest woman in the world retained the brainpower of those practically half her age.

Seven years ago, Myriam Marquez was driving home when she came to a four way stop. She wasn't far from her own driveway. She had stopped at this same intersection countless times. Yet she didn't know where she was.

"I called my daughter, panicked," Myriam says. A few excruciating minutes passed before she finally remembered where she was, and by that point she was sure she had Alzheimer's.

Her fears were soon validated. A battery of tests, including one for a gene that essentially guarantees Alzheimer's, confirmed her suspicions. She wasn't shocked; at least five of her father's siblings died with Alzheimer's symptoms. Two of her siblings have it, and her 47-year-old daughter is already beginning to show signs.

"I feel very blessed I'm still in the early stage," says Marquez, now 69 and living in Seattle. After her diagnosis, she charged into what she calls "warrior mode," campaigning to raise awareness of Alzheimer's while also working to stave off her own decline. Step one: Overhaul her "junk diet." Instead of pasta, pizza, and fast food, she now eats Mediterranean style, loading up on veggies; focusing on chicken, fish, and tofu for protein and limiting refined sugars and grains.

Dietary changes may seem inconsequential in the face of a diagnosis as monstrous as Alzheimer's, but there's reason to believe they're crucial. At a lab at Wake Forest School of Medicine, Suzanne Craft, a professor of gerontology and geriatric medicine, is studying how what we eat affects our brains and, in the process, revolutionizing the way we think about preventing and treating dementia.

Alzheimer's is the most common form of dementia and the National Institutes of Health's National Institute on Aging estimates that it's the sixth-leading cause of death in the United States. It often runs in families, but fewer than 5% of Alzheimer's cases are directly caused by a genetic variation such as the one Marquez carries. There's usually no way to tell who will get it--in part because no one really knows what causes it.

Today, most Alzheimer's research is based on the hypothesis that symptoms are triggered by abnormal deposits of proteins in the brain called amyloid plaques and tau tangles. With no confirmed cause and no effective long-term treatments for the disease, researchers have turned to other factors that might be at play. It's likely, says Laurie Ryan, chief of the Dementia of Aging Branch of the National Institute on Aging's division of neuroscience, that Alzheimer's does its damage via multiple pathways.

One of those pathways seems to involve type 2 diabetes. People who have it are at least twice as likely to develop Alzheimer's as those who don't – an association so strong that in 2005, neuropathologist named Suzanne de la Monte suggested that Alzheimer's could be referred to as "type 3 diabetes." That term, while controversial, has gained traction among some scientists as a way to focus attention on why the diseases often coexist.

Whatever you call it, the connection is worth exploring. Nearly 30 million Americans have diabetes, and 40% of people born today are expected to develop the disease in their lifetimes. If we want to protect America's mental health, we'd better figure out what the link is. Fast.

Ann Simpson is a vivacious woman with a cheerful smile and an easy laugh. Ask her about Alzheimer's though, and she quickly grows serious. "It's a nasty, nasty, disease," she says quietly.

Simpson, 69, has already lost her mother and one sister to the disease. Another sister has developed it as well. The sister living with Alzheimer's no longer remembers Ann's name or what money is. She ripped up a photo of a dear grandchild. "It's devastating," Simpson says, "and I'm scared to death that I may get it."

Given her family history, her deceased sister had both Alzheimer's and type 2 diabetes, Simpson was a perfect fit for a study led by Craft focusing on the role of insulin. Craft believes that much of the connection between Alzheimer's disease and type 2 diabetes has to do with this hormone.

Secreted in response to food, insulin removes sugar (glucose) from your blood and moves it into your cells, where it's used for energy. But sometimes the body doesn't use insulin as efficiently as it should. This is called insulin resistance, which means your body needs to release more insulin than normal to respond to the same amount of glucose. That might work for a while, but it's like using a leaky bucket to put out a fire. Because your body can pump out excess insulin for only so long, you'll eventually end up with chronically elevated blood sugar levels. That's type 2 diabetes.

The disease is well known for the havoc it wreaks on the body, but Craft and a growing number of researchers are more interested in what type 2 diabetes does to the brain. They're also exploring the role of insulin and blood sugar levels on memory in people who don't have diabetes, at least not yet. The No. 1 factor that affects your blood sugar levels and thus determines how much insulin you need, is your intake of carbohydrates.

The idea that there's a connection between diet and health may sound like old news, but Craft has gone beyond traditional observational studies.

"I'm an experimentalist by nature" she says, "and I wanted to do a very tightly controlled diet study to see whether we could affect people's cognition and the Alzheimer's markers in their spinal fluid by giving them a 'Western' diet high in sugar and saturated fat for 30 days."

That's exactly what she did. She took 49 older adults, 29 of whom had early signs of Alzheimer's disease and 20 of whom did not, and randomly assign them to one of two diets. The first, high in saturated fats and easily digested carbohydrates, was meant to mimic the stereotypical American diet. The second was more Mediterranean, with less saturated fat and a focus on complex carbs (like whole grains and legumes) that take a longer time to be absorbed and therefore don't cause the same spike in insulin as simple carbs do.

By the end of the month, the people who had been assigned to the Western-style diet performed worse on memory tests than they had at the beginning of the trial, and Alzheimer's -related beta-amyloid proteins showed up in their spinal fluid. Those who'd been assigned to the Mediterranean-style diet, on the other hand, did better on the tests, and their spinal fluid contained fewer Alzheimer's-related proteins. The effects reversed once participants returned to their normal eating patterns at the end of the study.

In a different trial, Craft found that people's cognitive abilities temporarily decreased-and that beta-amyloid in their spinal fluid temporarily increased-following a single high carb meal. "It's surprising to see changes in these markers after just one meal," says Ryan.

The question is "how does this happen?"

When Craft started her research on Alzheimer's some 20 years ago, she says "the idea that there was an important connection between insulin and the brain let alone insulin and Alzheimer's was viewed as so novel as to be fringe." Instead, researchers were focused on glucose. At the time, neurologists knew that the brains of people with Alzheimer's disease didn't use glucose properly. Craft designed a small trial that tested whether giving people a boost of glucose via a sugary beverage could temporarily improve their performance on a cognitive test. She was happy to find that it did. But it wasn't for the reason she had expected.

When the release of insulin was blocked, the memory benefit vanished. "The transient benefit to memory was tied not to the glucose but to elevations in insulin that happen naturally when people are given glucose," Craft says.

Scientists still don't understand why. But they do know that insulin is essential to the hippocampus, a seahorse-shaped structure in which our memories are created. Without adequate insulin, the hippocampus can't access the energy it needs to do its job and memories can't be recorded efficiently. Insulin also acts as a neurotransmitter, a chemical that enables brain cells to communicate with each other. It modulates the levels of other brain chemical that interact with memory. It also reduces inflammation, directs blood flow, and helps repair and create brain cells.

It might seem, therefore, that having extra insulin circulating in your body would be good for your mind. But that's not the case. When insulin levels in the body are abnormally high, the brain protects itself by restricting how much insulin it can absorb. In the short term, this shields the brain from the fluctuations in insulin levels that occur after meals. But when insulin levels are consistently elevated, as they are when you have insulin resistance, this process backfires and an insufficient amount of insulin reaches the brain. Ironically, the more insulin there is circulating in the bloodstream, the more likely it is that your brain isn't getting enough of it.

Craft isn't ready to say that less insulin in the brain actually causes Alzheimer's disease, in part because Alzheimer's is a highly specific term. Usually diagnosed after death, it means a person had the classic plaques and tangles as well as memory symptoms. And not everyone with age-related memory changes has Alzheimer's. "What we're studying is really the role of insulin in Alzheimer's symptoms," Craft says.

Craft and her team are now wrapping up a larger version of their original diet trial. She's also running a study she believes will prove that an ultra-low-carb diet is superior to the low-fat diet recommended by the American Heart Association when it comes to preserving brain health.

So far, Craft's findings offer a possible rationale for why a diet high in processed carbs (which promote insulin resistance) and type 2 diabetes (characterized by insulin resistance) increases the risk of Alzheimer's disease. They provide a plausible explanation for why several recent observational studies have found an association between a relatively low-carb, Mediterranean-inspired eating pattern called the MIND diet and a lower risk of Alzheimer's. Most important, they suggest that each of us can take steps to reduce our risk of developing Alzheimer's starting with our next meal.

Like any responsible scientist, Craft has caveats. Her studies are ongoing, and she doesn't yet know how powerful the effects of dietary patterns on Alzheimer's risk may be. There is no question, however that diet can affect our minds, and that the typical American diet doesn't appear to be healthy.

Other researchers are also cautiously optimistic. While these are preliminary findings, says Martha Clare Morris, a professor nutritional epidemiology at Rush University Medical Center who studies the role of diet in preventing chronic diseases like Alzheimer's, it's now an "aggressively studied area of research, as scientists and hopeful families alike clamor for a cure.

"People need to recognize that everything they put in their mouths has an impact on their brains," Craft explains. "Eating poorly and depriving your brain is absolutely going to affect how it functions over time."

She knows that some people will be skeptical. "Patients say to me, 'I ate well and exercised my whole life, and I'm 80 and I have Alzheimer's,'" Craft says. "What I say to them is that if you hadn't done that, you might have gotten Alzheimer's at 60."

Her Advice: Eat a Mediterranean-style diet featuring lots of produce and fatty fish. Avoid refined grains and processed foods. Exercise. "Diet and exercise work synergistically," Craft says. Basically, do everything in your power to avoid becoming insulin resistant.

"How diet works in the brain is complicated, but what to do is not," Craft says. "To a large extent, the health of our brains is under our control."

My Father died with Alzheimer's. It took him from us long before leukemia and its complications killed him.

The gene mentioned earlier in this article as a major susceptibility gene for Alzheimer's disease was discovered back in the 1990's. It's called APOE4. Inheritance of one APOE4 allele dose from Mom or Dad and the increase of our risk of getting Alzheimer's is tripled, and if we our 1-in-50 folks who have the APOE4 from both parents we may be at 9 times the risk. The highest frequency of APOE4 in the world is in Nigeria, but they also have some of the lowest Alzheimer's rates. To understand this paradox, one has to understand the role of APOE4. What does the APOE4 gene do? APOE4 is principal cholesterol carrier in the brain so their diet appeared to have trumped their genes. Their low cholesterol levels from their low intake of animal fat, living off of mainly grains and vegetables. High APOE4 with Alzheimer's is a rarity, thanks perhaps to the low cholesterol level which any of us can achieve by eating healthfully. These findings suggest that long term changes in plasma cholesterol can lead to changes in APOE4 gene expression. Just because you may have been dealt some bad genetic cards doesn't mean we can't reshuffle the deck with diet. We can't change our genetic makeup, but we can reduce or prevent high cholesterol.

In this study of a thousand people for over 20 years, APOE4 doubled the odds of Alzheimer's, but high cholesterol nearly tripled the threat, so the risk for Alzheimer's disease from treatable factors appears to be greater than that from the dreaded Alzheimer's susceptibility gene. In fact, projecting from their data controlling lifestyle factors could reduce a person's risk for Alzheimer's disease, even if they had the double barreled APOE4 gene from both parents, from 9 or 10 times the odds down to just 2.

People seem to have a fatalistic view about developing Alzheimer's disease, like if it's gonna happen it's gonna happen, but studies like this undermine such a view. We just need to emphasize the need for preventing and treating high blood pressure and cholesterol in the first place to reduce our risks for heart disease, strokes, and Alzheimer's disease and, as a result, potentially enhance quantity and quality of life. Of equal importance, these data should be comforting to anyone interested in reducing the risk for and future burden of Alzheimer's disease. (Sepehrnia et al., 1989)

India has the lowest rate of Alzheimer's. In rural Pennsylvania, the incidence rate of Alzheimer's disease among seniors is 19--19 people in a 1,000 over age 65 develop Alzheimer's every year in rural Pennsylvania. In rural India, using the same diagnostic criteria, that same rate is 3, confirming they have among the lowest reported Alzheimer's rates in the world. Although there isn't much to go on the lower prevalence of Alzheimer's in India is generally attributed to the turmeric consumption as part of curry. It's assumed that people who use turmeric regularly have a lower incidence of the disease. But let's not just assume. Of 1,000 people tested, those who consumed curry at least occasionally did do better on simple cognitive tests than those that didn't. Those that ate curry often had only about half the odds of showing cognitive impairment after adjusting for a wide variety of potential confounding factors. This suggest that curry consumption may be associated with better cognitive performance. It may be no coincidence that the country with among the lowest rates of Alzheimer's has among the lowest rates of meat consumption, with a significant chunk of the population eating meat-free and egg-free diets. We've known for over 20 years now that those who eat meat, red meat or white meat, appear between 2 to 3 times more likely to become demented compared to vegetarians. And the longer one eats meat-free the lower the associated risk of dementia.

TREATING ALZHEIMER'S WITH TURMERIC

An exciting case series was published in 2012. Three Alzheimer's patients treated with turmeric and their symptoms declined, along with the burden on their caregivers. What that means in real life!

Case#1: an 83-year old woman started losing her memory becoming disoriented. Then she started having problems taking care of herself, wandering aimlessly, incontinent. And after the turmeric, her agitation, apathy, anxiety and irritability were relieved. She had less accidents. Furthermore, she began to laugh again and sing again and knit again. After taking turmeric for more than a year, she came to recognize her family, and now lives a peaceful life without a significant behavioral or psychological symptom of dementia

Case#2: was similar, but with hallucinations and delusions and depression, which appeared relieved by turmeric. She began to recognize her family again and now lives in a peacefully serene manner. And the third case, similar as well, including an improvement in cognition.

The first demonstration that turmeric may be effective and safe for the treatment of the behavioral and psychological symptoms of dementia in Alzheimer's disease patients. They call it a drug, but it's just a spice. You can walk into any grocery store and buy it for a few bucks. They were giving people like a teaspoon a day which comes out to be about 15 cents.

Two trials using curcumin supplements rather than turmeric, however, failed to show a benefit. Curcumin is just one of hundreds of phytochemicals found in turmeric. Concentrated into pill form at up to 40 times the dose, no evidence of efficacy was found. Why didn't they get the same dramatic results we saw in the three case reports? Well those three cases may have been total flutes but on the other hand, turmeric, the whole food, is greater than the sum of its parts.

There's a long list of compounds that have been isolated from turmeric and it's possible that each component in the mixture of curcumin-like compounds plays a distinct role in making it useful in Alzheimer's disease, hence a mixture of compounds might better represent turmeric and its medicinal value better than curcumin alone. But why concoct some artificial mixture when Mother Nature already did it for us with turmeric? Because you can't patent the spice, and if you can't patent it, how are you going to charge more than 15 cents?

Recommend the video series "Awakening from Alzheimer's" by Peggy Sarlin a 12 video series, with 12 Alzheimer's specialist One is Dr. Richard Brown a clinical psychiatrist at Columbia an expert in supplements for dementia and Alzheimer's. Dr. Brown treats other Doctors and teaches them the effectiveness of supplements for treating mental decline one doctor claimed his mental clarity improved by 20 years.

Saffron Dr. Brown recommends the brand "Optimize Saffron" from the Life Extension Foundation. One tablet with breakfast and another with dinner. He emphasizes being careful about purity and avoid Chines manufactured supplements and list several manufactures who operate with pharmaceutical standards. In a 22 week, multicenter, randomized, double-blind controlled trial of (saffron) in the treatment of mild-to-moderate Alzheimer's disease. Saffron versus Aricept, the leading drug. Saffron worked as well as Aricept which just slows down the progression. Dr. Brown believes saffron pulls amyloid out of the brain, reduces craving for carbohydrates and is a powerful anti-oxidant.

Another Doctor in the series discussed the importance of sleep he has a website, what else thesleepdoctor.com. His advice best time to go to bed 10:30, sleep seven and a half hours be consistent get up at the same time every day.

Homocysteine is considered a strong, independent risk factor for the development of dementia and Alzheimer's disease. Having a blood level over 14 may double our risk in the Framingham Study, they estimated that as many as 1 in 6 Alzheimer's cases may be attributable to elevated homocysteine in the blood-now thought to play a role in brain damage, and cognitive and memory decline. Our body can detoxify homocysteine, though, using three vitamins-folate, vitamin B12 and vitamin B6.

A double-blind randomized controlled trial found that homocysteine-lowering by B vitamins can slow the rate of accelerated brain atrophy in people with mild cognitive impairment. As we age, our brain slowly atrophies, but the shrinking is much accelerated in patients from Alzheimer's disease. An intermittent rate of shrinkage is found in people with mild cognitive impairment. The thinking is that maybe if we could slow the rate of brain loss, we could slow the conversion to Alzheimer's disease. They tried giving people B vitamins for two years and they found it markedly slowed the rate of brain shrinkage. The rate of atrophy in those with high homocysteine levels was cut in half. A simple, safe treatment can slow the accelerated rate of brain loss.

A follow up study went further by demonstrating that B vitamin treatment reduces, by as much as sevenfold, the brain atrophy in the regions specifically vulnerable to the Alzheimer's disease process.

The beneficial effect of B vitamins was confined to those with high homocysteine, indicating a relative deficiency in one of those three vitamins. So, wouldn't it be better to not get deficient in the first place? Most people get enough B12 and B6, but the reason these folks were stuck up at a homocysteine of 11 is that they probably weren't getting enough folate, which is found predominantly in beans and greens. 96% of Americans don't even make the minimum recommended amount of dark green leafy vegetables, the same pitiful number who don't eat the minimum recommendation for beans.

If you put people on a healthy diet, a plant-based diet, you can drop their homocysteine levels 20% in just one week up from around 11 down to 9. The fact that they showed significant homocysteine lowering without any pills, without supplements- even at one week suggests that multiple mechanisms may have been at work. They suggest it may be because of the fiber. Every gram of daily fiber consumption may increase folate levels in the blood nearly 2% perhaps by boosting vitamin production in our colon by our friendly gut bacteria. It also could be from the decreased methionine intake; that's where homocysteine comes from. Homocysteine is a breakdown product of methionine, which comes mostly from animal protein. Thus decreased methionine intake on a plant-based diet may be another factor contributing too lower, safer homocysteine levels.

The irony is that those who eat plant-based diets long term, have terrible homocysteine levels. Meat eaters up at 11 but vegetarians at nearly 14 and vegans at 16. They get plenty of fiber and folate, but they're not getting enough vitamin B12. But add vitamin B12 or eating vitamin B12 fortified foods the vegan homocysteine can drop below 5.

Mounting evidence indicates that Alzheimer's Disease is primarily a vascular disorder impaired circulation in the brain. Vascular risk factors, such as high cholesterol, can be thought of as a ticking time bomb to Alzheimer's Disease. What's bad for the heart may be bad for the mind.

Autopsy studies have found that Alzheimer's brains have significantly more cholesterol than normal brains, and it specifically appears to accumulate in the Alzheimer brain plaques. In addition, having high cholesterol may even damage the blood brain barrier into the brain. So, a high-fat diet may not only increase cholesterol levels in the blood, but also the influx of cholesterol into the central nervous system. Individuals with higher cholesterol levels at midlife have a higher risk of going on to develop Alzheimer's disease. Cholesterol over 250 could potentially triple the odds of Alzheimer's.

High-tech PET scanning of the brain can directly correlate the amount of so-called bad cholesterol in our blood with the amount of amyloid build up in our brains. You can do it right in a Petri dish. Adding cholesterol makes them churn out more the amyloid that makes up Alzheimer plaques, whereas removing cholesterol can decrease the levels of amyloid released from the cells and amyloid degradation is less efficient in a high cholesterol environment.

Once in the brain, cholesterol can also undergo auto-oxidation, causing the formation of highly toxic free radicals so they may also directly affect neurodegeneration within the brain. (de la TORRE, 2002)

Every 70 seconds another American is diagnosed with Alzheimer's. The best science we have for prevention is a whole food plant base diet, exercise at least 40 minutes every day (aerobic exercise forcing oxygen to the brain) getting seven and a half hours of sleep and to continually challenge your brain; learn a second language, play crossword puzzles, watch documentaries, be creative write a book.

Dr. David L Katz, director of Yale's Research Prevention Center, believes that Alzheimer's is 80% preventable. He goes on to explain there are two theoretical and one empirical. The two theoreticals have growing evidence one being insulin resistance (type three diabetes) and vascular disease (clogged arteries). The empirical evidence are the blue zones. People who live the longest lives on earth rarely contracting dementia or Alzheimer's.

LONGEVITY

(USDA) dietary guidelines recommend that most people need to choose meals or snacks that are high in nutrients but low-to-moderate in energy content and that doing so "offers reduction of risk for a number of chronic diseases that are major public health problems."

Well, they're talking about fruits and vegetables - so what would happen if a population centered their entire diet around vegetables they might end up living the longest lives in the world.

Okinawans are, one of the longest living cultures on earth one of the so called blue zones. We know what they ate because Okinawa was governed by the U.S. Military after WWII until control was returned to Japan in the late '72. The traditional Okinawa diet only 1percent fish 1 percent meat same with dairy and eggs so it was 96 percent plant based and 90 percent whole food plant based centered around purple and orange potatoes. Nathan Pritikin would applaud them.

What if you ate 100 percent whole food plant based diet? You would have to go to Loma Linda California and study the Adventist part of their teachings which is not to smoke or drink and not to eat animal products. Like Baptists who are taught not to drink or smoke, you have people who comply and those who don't. But back to longevity--the ones who ate 100 percent whole food and lived a healthy, active lifestyle lived on average 9 years longer than the average American. Interestingly, those who were flexitarian eating an oz of nuts a day lived longer than the vegans who didn't eat nuts but not as long as the whole food diet who also ate nuts and a healthy lifestyle.

Today the Okinawans longevity is history. They have 15 KFC among the array of fast food outlets and once the thinnest people of Japan now are the heaviest. One Japanese health official quipped, "it's time for the Okinawans to eat the Okinawan diet."

Dr. Joel Fuhrman, New York times best-selling author of "Eat to Live" talked about one of his patients. His name was Jack. He was in his early 60's when he first visited Dr. Fuhrman's office. He had the typical chronic American diseases: High Blood pressure, High cholesterol, High Blood sugar. Now Jack is 92. He doesn't take any of the medication that he needed when he was in his 60's. He earned his health back. "I was playing singles tennis with him a couple of weeks ago and he was jumping around like a jack rabbit." I thought that was a worthy goal.

In 1999 a theoretical high energy physicist from Los Alamos joined up with two biologists to define Universal scaling laws that apply across the board. Any clinical implications? The number of heartbeats are remarkably similar whether you're a hamster or a whale. Even though a mouse lives only a couple of years, their heartrate beats 500 to 600 times a minute. Whereas the heartbeat of a Galapagos Tortoise beats 100 times slower and they live 100 times longer. There is such a remarkable consistence. A provocative observation! Can human life be extended by cardiac slowing?

If humans are predetermined to have about 3 billion heart beats would a reduction in resting heart rate extend life? This is not just some academic question one might estimate that a reduction in mean heart rate, resting heart rate from 70 to 60 (which many athletes have) would increase life span from 80 to 93.3 years.

From the evidence accumulated so far, a high resting heart rate is associated with an increase in cardiovascular and all-cause mortality in the general population, as well as in hypertensive patients, patients with diabetes, patients with stable coronary heart disease or those with stemi. So faster resting heart rate are associated with shorter life expectancies.

Higher levels of resting heart rate (HR) have been associated with Sudden Cardiac Death (SCD) This has been proven as a risk factor not a risk marker. The conclusion from 12 coharts, 112,000 men and women resting heart rates of above 65 beats/min has a strong independent effect on premature mortality. You can take your heart rate right now one beat a second is ideal. Don't worry if it's too fast. Heart rate is modifiable. There are drugs and lifestyle regimes to reduce heart rate.

Men with no evidence of ischemic heart disease and HR of 90 beats/min had 5 times higher risk of SCD compared to men with a rate of 60 beats a minute. So the first symptom is your last! A rate of 90 is a similar risk as smoking. This is particularly important to diabetics. Having a high resting heart rate puts you at the same risk as the general public but you have a greater risk of new onset of progressive nephropathy and retinopathy.

The accepted rate of heartbeat has long been 60-100. What was the science behind that? None. It was adapted as a matter of convenience because it fit on the squares of EKG paper. Amazing.

A group of men and woman performed aerobic exercise for 12 weeks lowered their heart rate 3 points. Eating one cup of cooked beans, chickpeas, or lentils for 12 weeks lowered the heart rate 3.4 points and it lowers A1C from 7.4 to 6.9, so eat your pulses for you pulse.

Researchers have been demonstrating for more than 80 years that restricting the food intake of animals ranging from one-celled creatures to humans results in a lengthened life-span. Unrestricted feeding, on the other hand, promotes increased rate of growth, a greater amount of body fat, earlier onset of degenerative diseases, and premature death. Not only the quantity of food but its composition affects the aging process.

My niece Amanda, a remarkable young woman, had a rough time raising her two young sons while her husband, Chris, a top sergeant in a National Guard combat engineering company was deployed to Iraq and Afghanistan. They removed 1500 IEDs think Hurt Locker. Two of Chris's young combat qualified soldiers had heart attacks.

After Amanda's sons were older, she enrolled in nursing school graduated top in her class. Amanda is the kind of nurse you want- a tireless advocate for her patients. Her professionalism, attitude, ability, and devotion did not go unnoticed by the hospital promoting her to head nurse waving the time requirement. When I mentioned I was writing this book she sent me this text.

A 24-year-old African American, diabetic, comes to hospital at least once a month. Blood sugar on arrival is anywhere between 500-900. He is not compliant with diabetic diet and the doctor says he will not live to 30. "You can't get a blood sample from his arm. You just get this yellow fat and cholesterol." Maybe one diabetic death a week. This is one of two hospitals in a small city of 70,000. She says maybe because she only works 14-hours-a-day 4 days a week, she does not know what happens the other 3 days. In other words, it's so common it's not conversational.

America has a childhood obesity epidemic which means we have a childhood diabetes epidemic. Children with diabetes have a 20-year shorter lifespan   It's your choice!

In 2010, the chair of the nutrition department at Loma Linda University published a paper suggesting that giving up meat entirely is an effective way to combat childhood obesity, pointing to population studies demonstrating that people eating plant-based diets are consistently thinner than those who eat meat.

THE HISPANIC PARADOX: WHY DO LATINOS LIVE LONGER?

Hispanics living in the United States have less education, a higher poverty rate and less access to health care than non-Hispanic whites. Hispanics living in the US represent the ultimate paradigm of healthcare disparities. With the highest rate of uninsured people, the lowest rates of screening for hypercholesterolemia, hypertension, and other cvds risk factors, with the lowest rates of smoking counseling and with the poorest levels of blood pressure control, glycemic control, and other measures of deficient quality of care so Latinos living in the US should have dismal health statistics.

According to the latest public health data the life expectance of white men and women was 76.4 for men and 81.1 for women, lives of black men and women cut short by years men 71.6 women 77.8. How do Hispanics do amazingly they beat out everyone men 78.9 and females 81.1

Hispanics had a 24% lower risk of all-cause mortality and lower risks of nine of the leading 15 causes of death in the USA (cancer and heart disease).

After debate this fact was concluded as true instead of dismissing it maybe this represents a major opportunity to identify a protective factor for CVD applicable to the rest of the population.

The foreign-born Hispanic mortality advantage erased for U.S.-born Hispanics? Negative acculturation may deteriorate the positive health behaviors among Hispanic immigrants over time and across generations, thereby eliminating the initial Hispanic mortality advantage

They didn't exercise more they did smoke less but that was factored into the data. Must be their diet although Hispanic represented approximately 11 percent of the population, they accounted for 33 percent of all cooked dry edible bean consumption. Eating 4 or 5 pounds a month opposed to 4 or 5 pounds a year. That may help explain the Hispanic paradox a diet rich in legumes and are very high in fiber and have recently been shown to attenuate systemic inflammation significantly reducing the risk of various cancers which Hispanics have less of and have a better survival rate. They also eat more corn, tomatoes, rice and chill peppers. Looking at cancer rates around the world bean consumption was associated with lower rates of colon, breast and prostate cancers and so was rice and corn.

The Hispanics eat 5 or 6 servings of fruits and vegetables a day not meeting the recommended 9 and they have less heart attacks but it's still the number one killer of Hispanics in the USA so maybe they should eat more fruits and vegetables.

Earl Reece Stadtman (1919-2008) One of America's most notable biochemist Chief of the Laboratory of Biochemistry at the Nation Heart Institute and also a member of the National Academy of Sciences. "Aging is a disease. The human lifespan simply reflects the level of free radical damage that accumulates in cells. When enough damage accumulates cells can't survive properly anymore and they just simple give up." (Harman, 1972). The Biologic Clock: The Mitochondria? It's the loss of cellular activity in the mitochondria. Mitochondria are like miniature blast furnaces inside your cells where the food that we eat is converted into usable energy. It's here that inside these fireworks an oxygen molecule can be transformed into what is called a super oxide which can damage our delicate cellular machinery basically we're rusting that's what oxidation is ageing is the slow oxidation of our body. Oxidative stress is why we get wrinkles why we loss some of our memory why our organs systems break down as we get older. How do we slow down our oxidation. By eating foods that contain antioxidants. How do you keep your fruit salad from turning brown add lemon juice which has vitamin c and antioxidant which can keep your food from oxidizing it can do the same thing inside our body. Many antioxidants can't penetrate the mitochondria membrane so they protect our dna and other cells but that's why our bodies have an enzyme called superoxide dismutase it's a detoxifying enzyme within our mitochondria that neutralizes super oxide turns it back into oxygen. Because of its role it's considered a tumor suppressor staving off cancer it's consider neuroprotective in our brain staving off dementia. This has become so accepted by the scientific community. That a paper was written asking the question is their anymore to aging at all. The question is how do we boast the enzyme activity of this antiaging anticancer, anti-Alzheimer's enzyme. Become a vegetarian last year researchers compared this enzymes activity between omnivores vs vegetarians eating vegetarian seem to boast this enzymes activity 300 percent. No wonder vegetarians live longer no wonder they have less cancer, less vascular disease.

A higher gene expression in vegetarians thus a better defense against superoxide radicals might be expected as a consequence of a vegetarian diet. The higher protection against chronic diseases in vegetarians may be explained by both epigenetic and chemico-physiolgical aspects. You think you are born with genes and are just stuck with them we now know what we eat can change gene expression. In this case eating vegetarian seems to boast the activity of one the most important enzymes in the body. (Harman, 1972)

Amla Indian gooseberries arguably the most important medicinal plant in Ayuredic medicine, and also used in traditional Chinese and Thai medicine. Pre-clinical studies have evidently shown that amla possesses anti-fever properties, anti-pain, anti-cough, anti-clogging, anti-stress, heart protective, stomach protecting, anti-anemia, anti-cancer, anti-cholesterol, wound healing, anti-diarrhea, as well as protecting the liver, kidneys and nerves. It can evidently be used as a snake venom neutralizer, as well as hair tonic. A friend that I garden with, a professor at the University and originally from India, suggested I try it. Additional studies have shown it lowers blood sugar but it's antioxidant properties is what impressed me one teaspoon of amla in a fruit smoothie is more antioxidant than most American get in a week. It tastes terrible but it's not noticeable in a smoothie.

OBSERVATIONS

The American Medical Association has given up on weight control for the American public because the diets they recommended didn't work so now they focus on metabolic control. With diabetes, it's blood sugar; with atherosclerosis, it's cholesterol control; and with hypertension, it's blood pressure medication. None of these approaches are treating the disease. They are treating symptoms of these diseases. It's not really their fault. They are not taught nutrition in medical school. Amazing.

The American Journal of Nutrition did a study for doctors and their patients, simple true or false questions on nutrition. Who scored better? The patients. Yet we assume they know and in reality you, the person on the street, know more. Big Pharma runs our medical system. They pay for the research that's taught in our medical schools that promote their drugs. 106,000 American die every year from what's called ARD (Adverse Reaction to Drugs) -- not overdose, not the wrong drug, it's the drug prescribed, and the body says "nope" and you're dead. Which contributes to medical care being the third leading cause of death in America, after heart disease and cancer.

Don't misunderstand me I'm all for research and advanced treatment but when over 80% of the chronic disease could be prevented. Dr. Burkett put it this way early diagnosis and treatment never prevented a disease. He also said big hospital means poor community health and small stools. He was big on eating lots of fiber.

"Willpower" There is an unspoken assumption that some problems require "X" amount of willpower to master, and if we don't quite have "X" amount then we may be doomed to fail. For decades, therapists and counselors have accepted this tacit assumption-that a person's "willpower" is essentially a fixed quantity within us that varies from person to person. Some people seem to have great ability to withstand temptations, where others seem to struggle much more.

However, in the past decade, a series of investigations into willpower uncovered an astonishing fact: Willpower is not a fixed quantity within individuals. A person's willpower varies enormously from hour to hour, depending upon the degree of immediately recent mental stress. Specifically, mental stress (decision making) causes a decision-area of the brain becomes glucose-depleted, and thus fatigued. At that point, the individual is experiencing "decision fatigue" and is becoming increasingly impulsive. Willpower is actually brain glucose. Studies led by social psychologist Roy Baumeister and his colleagues have left no doubt about it-when your mind is working extra hard for even ten minutes, you becoming mentally fatigued and your willpower gets shaky.

So what can we do about this?

There are four simple, effective fundamental strategies for supporting your willpower. They are:

1) Cleaning your room

2) Eating something healthy first

3) Daily exercise

4) Getting to bed on time

These sound ridiculously low tech and unimaginative. However, each is fitting a piece of the willpower puzzle together. Keeping a tidy home environment means that your mind has less worries about what you "should" be doing, than if you keep looking at a stack of messy paper on table and desks. A tidy environment will deplete your willpower less than a messy one, and thus help you with other goals requiring your limited willpower, such as healthy eating and living choices. When feeling a bit stressed and even a little mentally fatigued, we often desire to eat something sugary, eat something healthy first. Foods with some substance-such as complex carbohydrates (like a banana or some oatmeal or a bean burrito) will support your brain glucose much more effectively. These foods are more slowly digested than junk food, cause a gentle but steady blood glucose rise, and support your brain for a long steady ride. Next, some modest daily exercise routine will also support your willpower. This routine can often be very simple, like taking 10 minutes a day in your own place, dancing to some favorite music. There is no need to go to the gym and make a big production out of this. I simply jump rope for about ten minutes and get a great workout. Keep it simple if you need to, if working out isn't your thing. A modest program is a key component of willpower support. It is not yet known why exercise has been shown to successfully support willpower, but it could be that exercise helps the body more effectively release glucose from storage on demand, and thus helps you be more resilient when under stress. So get moving but it's fine if you keep it simple.

Finally, shut off the electronic toys and get to sleep! It has recently been shown why sleep is so important: Is during sleep that the brain does it's housekeeping, literally cleaning itself up. When short of sleep, our minds are literally working against yesterday's mental debris, and we deprive our minds of their full power, and that includes our willpower.

Healthy food, exercise, sleep and an orderly environment may not sound fancy, but they are the fundamentals of supporting your mind. Treat your mind well, and it will stick by you and help you when you need it most. And that is how you can begin and exciting new path toward becoming healthier happier, and having the life you deserve.

Douglas Lisle, PhD Director of Research for True North Health Center and author of The Pleasure Trap

THE TELOMERE EFFECT

Preventive Medicine Column

January 6, 2017

Listen to Your Telomeres

One of the reasons cardiology tends to advance so rapidly compared to other medical disciplines- with very noteworthy benefits, such as marked declines in both premature death and disability related to heart disease- is because of the power of surrogate markers. Surrogate markers in medicine are generally things we can measure in the short term that tell us with at least reasonable, and sometimes excellent, fidelity about likely outcomes in the long term. Cardiology's cup is full to the brim with good surrogate markers, such as LDL cholesterol, blood pressure, and heart rate.

We should distinguish, however, the value of surrogate markers from what we might call "duplicative markers." Just because we can measure something doesn't mean there is always much value in doing so.

In medicine, we rely at times on technology to tell us what we already know. Consider, for instance, the burgeoning array of studies using some cutting edge technology, like fMRI, to study brain responses to food. You already know that when you eat, say,

French fries, you experience intense but probably rather fleeting pleasure. Do we really need cutting edge technology to show us changes in metabolic activity in the pleasure center of our brain to tell us we found something...pleasurable?

Surrogate markers are different, because they tell us something we otherwise couldn't know unless we waited for the outcomes they predict, and then-it would be too late. It's not helpful to find out after a heart attack that we are at risk for heart disease, for instance. It's even less helpful to find out after we die that our life expectancy isn't everything we might wish.

Imagine, then, if we had a surrogate marker for healthy life expectancy itself. Imagine how powerful it would be if something we could measure that changed rapidly in response to influences both good and bad, reliably predicted the length of healthy life. That would be quite a boon, since otherwise, the only way to show changes in the length of life would require waiting lifetimes. I suspect we can all agree it would be something of an anti-climax to learn only on your hundredth birthday that you were likely to live to 100.

It turns out, there is just such a surrogate marker for the length of life. Telomeres are, structurally, caps at the ends of our chromosomes- they have been compared to the plastic caps at the ends of shoelaces. Health-promoting exposures, or alternatively the slings and arrows of outrageous fortune, can lengthen or shorten telomeres, respectively. The length of telomeres, in turn, predicts the length of healthy life.

Not perfectly, of course; even with gloriously long telomeres, it would be imprudent to stand in the path of a moving train. But powerfully. Imagine, then, how great it would be if we could talk directly to our telomeres, and find out how they're doing.

Now, we can. In a newly released book called The Telomere Effect, two leading experts, one of them a Nobel Prize winner, go carefully through the science enumerating the effects of diverse exposures on telomere length and function. Drs. Elizabeth Blackburn and Elissa Epel proceed study by study, and cover everything from stress to diet, exercise to sleep, the influences of environment when we are just in the womb to those of social interactions throughout life. They then translate each cluster of studies into practical tips you can apply.

If telomeres could talk, and tell us what makes them lengthen or shrink, what makes them happy or unhappy, they would provide us compelling, powerful, actionable intelligence and a measure of control over our longevity. Conversing with telomeres would be the next best thing to sipping from the fountain of youth.

The length of telomeres is predictive of the length of healthy life, while providing the lead-time necessary to do something about it. And, in fact, they are not just markers of health span, but actual mechanisms of it; vital telomeres transmit that vitality to the cells in which they reside. Drs. Blackburn and Epel speak up for telomeres, and provide guidance in nurturing that very vitality.

Of course, the lifestyle prescription that's good for our telomeres is one we already knew was good for us in general. But a vivid view of aging itself at the cellular level that does not require years and decades to elapse is a rarefied vista indeed, a truly unique window of opportunity. This book opens that window to us all.

If only telomeres could talk to us, they would provide unique insights into human aging, with the time to do something about it. It turns out they can, in the authoritative voices of Drs. Blackburn and Epel, on the pages of The Telomere Effect. Telomeres are talking now; I think everyone should listen.

-fin   Dr. David L. Katz; www.davidkatzmd.com; founder, True Health Initiative

Drs. Blackburn and Epel in The Telomere Effect reveal what shortens our Telomeres and what we can do to preserve and lengthen our Telomeres the so called life's fuse. This is a revolutionary approach to living younger, healthier, and longer. I recommend this book to everyone who has Telomeres.

What shortens Telomeres the usual suspects the standard American diet, stress, excess Alcohol, abusive relations, living in a dangerous neighborhood lack of quality sleep, lack of exercise, insulin resistance, inflammation, pesticides, chemical exposure and depression to name a few.

Some things that preserve and lengthens our Telomeres whole plant based diet with adequate amount of omega-3 fatty acids (DHA, EPA) vitamin D3 exercise people who exercised regularly had Telomeres 16 years younger than couch potatoes. Mindfulness and yoga one style of yoga Kirtan Kriya was used in a study at UCLA. Caregivers who had mild depression practiced Kirtan Kriya for twelve minutes a day for two months, they increased their telomerase by 43 percent and decreased their gene expression related to inflammation. (A control group listened to relaxing music; their telomerase increased, too, but only by 3.7. percent. Telomerase is the enzyme that replenishes telomeres.

The Telomere Effect is comprehensive what you would expect from a Nobel Prize winner.

MIND-BODY CONNECTION

The Chinese 3000 years ago thought it so important they guarded it as a state secret. There's a nerve, called the vagus nerve, that goes directly from our brain to our chest to our stomach, and connects our brain back and forth to our heart and our gut, and even our immune system. The vagus nerve is like the hardwiring that allows our brain to turn down inflammation within our body. When you hear about the mind-body connection-that's what the vagus nerve is, and does. So, there's been "increasing interest in treating a wide range of disorders with implanted devices for stimulating ...vagus (nerve) pathways. Certain eastern traditionslike "Yoga, QIGong, an Zen" figured a way to do it without having electrodes implanted.

A healthy heart is not a metronome. Your heart rate goes up and down with your breathing. When you breathe in, your heart rate tends to go up. When you breathe out, your heart rate tends to go down." Test it out on yourself right now by feeling your pulse change as you breathe in and out.

That heart rate variability is a measure of vagal tone-the activity of your vagus nerve. Now there's a whole other oscillating cycle going on at the same time that's speeding, then slowing, your heart rate based on moment-to-moment changes in your blood pressure.The physics tell you "all oscillating feedback systems with a constant delay have the characteristic of resonance"-meaning you can boost the amplitude if you get the cycles in sync. So, if you breathe in at just the right frequency, you can force the cycles in sync, and boost your heart rate variability. Why would we do this? Practicing slow breathing a few minutes a day may have lasting beneficial effects on a number of medical and emotional disorders including asthma, irritable bowel syndrome, fibromyalgia, and depression. You can use this technique to significantly drop your blood pressure within minutes. The hope is if you practice this a few minutes a day, you can have long-lasting effects the rest of the day, breathing normally.

Do What? Slow breathing, five or six breaths per minute, split equally between breathing in and breathing out should do it. So, like, five seconds in, then five seconds out, all the while breathing "shallowly and naturally"—you don't want to hyperventilate. Natural shallow breaths, but just breathing really slowly.

Mindfulness and Meditation being in the moment not thinking about the past or future but the present where you actually live mindful is helpful when you start to get a snack ask yourself am I hungry be mindful or ask yourself is this healthy it can be that simply. (PubMed, Matter over mind source and nutritionfacts. Org Greger)

EXERCISE IS MEDICINE

Nathan Pritikin advocated 50 years ago for everyone to walk at a brisk pace for an hour a day or two 30 or 3 20 minute sessions. The World Health Organization recommended an hour a day of walking. What does the science show 90 minutes a day of moderate intensity exercise such as walking at a pace you breathe through your mouth (you can carry on a conversation but you could not sing) or 40 minutes of vigorous exercise a day. We have irrefutable evidence that exercise is necessary for a healthy life. Not walking a minimum of an hour a day is now considered a health risk equivalent to smoking, being obese or heavy drinking. You should walk after each meal as it lowers blood sugar. Meta-analysis of physical activity dose and longevity found that the equivalent of about an hour a day of brisk (4mph) was good but 90 minutes was even better. An hour long walk each day may reduce mortality by 24 percent. I mention walking because it's an exercise nearly everyone can do. Aerobic exercise is not enough.

Sarcopenia (from the Greek sarx for flesh and penia for loss) is the age-associated loss of muscle mass and function. Sarcopenia is determined by two factors: the initial amount of muscle mass and the rate at which it declines with age. The rate of muscle loss with age appears to be fairly consistent, approximately 1%-2% per year past the age of 50 years. Age related insulin resistance may contribute the chemistry and metabolic functions aren't clear but regular exercise, particularly weight training, is essential for preserving and increasing muscle mass. In addition to building muscle, strength training promotes mobility, enhances fitness, and improves bone health. A recent study in Japan with older men who were informed of the loss of muscle mass reversed the decline and added muscle so it's a choice.

MODERATE-INTENSITY ACTIVITIES

Bicycling, canoeing, downhill skiing, dancing, hiking, housework, skating, shooting baskets, jumping on a trampoline, playing Frisbee, swimming recreationally, tennis doubles, walking briskly 4 mph, yard work and yoga

VIGOROUS ACTIVITIES

Backpacking, basketball, bicycling uphill, circuit weight training, cross-country skiing, jogging, jumping jacks, jumping rope, push-ups and pull-ups, racquetball, running, scuba diving, tennis (singles) squash, step aerobics, swimming laps, walking briskly uphill

SITTING--THE NEW SMOKING

A recent review of 43 studies analyzing daily activity and cancer rates found that people who reported sitting for more hours of the day had a 24% greater risk of developing colon cancer, a 32% higher risk of lung cancer regardless of how much they exercised. In another study involving a group of men and women who reported exercising the same amount, each additional hour they spent sitting was linked to a drop in their fitness level. In other words, sitting was chipping away at some of the benefits of exercise. Suggestions include getting a standing desk burning 500 to 1000 additional calories a day or a treadmill desk. Why is sitting around so bad for you? One reason may be endothelial dysfunction, the inability of the inner lining of your blood vessels to signal your arteries to relax normally in response to blood flow. Just as your muscles atrophy if you don't use them, "use it or lose it" may apply to arterial function as well. Increased blood flow promotes a healthy endothelium. Blood flow is what maintains the stability and integrity of the inner lining of your arteries. Without the constant tugging flow with each heartbeat of exertion, you can end up a sitting duck for arterial dysfunction diseases. If your office can't accommodate a standing desk, there is preliminary evidence from observational and interventional studies which suggest that regular interruptions in sitting time can be beneficial. And they don't have to be long. Breaks could be as short as one minute and not necessarily entail strenuous exercise-- just walking up and down stairs may be enough.

What if you have a sitting job in which you can't take frequent breaks, like truck driving? Is there any way to improve your endothelial function sitting on your butt? Diet-wise drinking green tea every two hours can help keep your endothelium functional, as can eating meals with greens and other nitrate-rich vegetables.

Turmeric may also help. One head-to-head study found that daily ingestion of the turmeric component curcumin can improve endothelial function just as well as up to an hour a day of aerobic exercise. You still need to move around as much as possible the combination of turmeric and exercise appears to work even better than either option alone.

OPTIMIZING RECOVERY

Anyone who works out regularly knows about sore muscles. Burning sensation during strenuous exercise, which may be related to the buildup of lactic acid in your muscles, and then there's delayed-onset muscle soreness, the kind you get in the days following extreme physical activity. Delayed soreness is likely the result of inflammation caused by micro tears in your muscles and can adversely affect athletic performance in the days following a heavy workout. If you're suffering from an inflammatory reaction, the bioflavonoids in citrus can help with the lactic acid buildup, and you may need to ramp up the anthocyanin flavonoids in berries to deal with the inflammation.

Muscle biopsies of athletes have confirmed that eating blueberries, for example, can significantly reduce exercise-induced inflammation. Studies using cherries show that this anti-inflammation effect can translate into faster recovery time, reducing the strength loss from excessive bicep curling from 22 percent down to only 4 percent in male college students over the subsequent four days. The muscle-soothing effects of berries don't only work for weight lifters; follow-up studies have shown that cherries can also help reduce muscle pain in long-distance runners and aid in recovery from marathons.

Eating two cups of watermelon prior to intense physical activity was found to significantly reduce muscle soreness.

PREVENTING EXERCISE-INDUCED OXIDATIVE STRESS

Studies have demonstrated that ultra-marathoners show evidence of DNA damage in about 10 percent of their cells tested during and up to two weeks following a race. But most of us aren't ultra-marathoners.

Might short bouts of exercise still damage your DNA? Yes. After just five minutes of moderate or intense cycling, you can get an uptick in DNA damage. What about using antioxidant-rich foods to douse the free radicals? Researchers led subjects onto treadmills and cranked up the intensity until they nearly collapsed. While a spike in free-radical levels was witnessed in the control group, subjects who loaded up on watercress two hours before exercising actually ended up with fewer free radicals after the treadmill test than when they started. After two months of eating a daily serving of watercress, no DNA damage resulted, no matter how much it seemed the subjects were punished on the treadmill. So with a healthy diet, you can get the best of both worlds—all the benefits of strenuous exercise without excess free-radical damage. As a review in the Journal of Sports Sciences put it, those who eat plant-based diets may naturally "have an enhance antioxidant defense system to counter exercise-induced oxidative stress. Whether it's about training longer or living longer, the science seems clear. Your quality and quantity of life improves when you eat a more plant based diet.

From the lost lectures of Nathan Pritikin: How important is exercise? We took a 20-year-old male, perfectly healthy, and put him in bed for 3 weeks. Afterward, he was only able to do 70% of his endurance on the treadmill, his blood values became abnormal, glucose went up, uric acid went up you lose calcium blood sends it out through your urine. Fortunately, it's possible through exercise to retain and increase bone density. We took two groups each of 15, 65-70 years old one group walked 1 hour a day 4 days a week while the other had no organized exercise. After a year the exercise group had no loss of skeleton weight the other group loss 9% of skeleton weight. Osteoporosis is an epidemic in this country. You will hear they didn't get enough calcium, drink enough milk but this is just a fable set up by the national dairy council. If you have a stroke victim with one arm paralyzed your blood flows too both. Bone density goes out through your urine. If you don't use it, you lose it. Also smoking reduces bone calcium but it's sucked up by your big Arora--not good.

EXERCISE FOR MORE CIRCULATION

New growth circulation gives you more blood flow so when you have narrow vessels or closed vessels you are able to pump enough blood to overcome the problem. Is this possible? The news is good in both animal studies and human studies. You can create new substantial blood flow even through you've blocked main arteries. We had a participant, an alumnus, who had an angiogram which showed both his femoral arteries were substantially closed. He had so little blood flow he could only walk a few hundred feet but every step would cause him great pain and he was in danger of course of developing gangrene and he came to our center. Here's a man who had cholesterol over 400 which we finally got his down over a period of time to below 200. It took him awhile to walk without pain but eventually he was able to walk 4 or 5 miles without pain. The amazing thing about this man, even though he had two closed femoral, he developed enough blood flow in his legs after two or three years to run a marathon 26 miles. Now everyday as a normal practice he runs 5 or 6 miles and when I talked to him just a short while ago, he said "I don't have any pain in my one leg at all when I run but in the other leg after about a mile I get a little pain it last about a mile then it disappears." So we've seen cases with the worst possible circulation re-establish circulation. One thing about exercise, if you're deficient in circulation you're going to improve your circulation.

In my long beach study back in 1975 we had about 15 or 18 men on my diet--the same one I recommend at my center for 5 months then there was another group of men who ate the regular American Diet. After 5 months we retested all on the treadmill. The men were selected all had insufficient circulation in their legs. When they started the average man could only walk 200 ft. and after that he had to stop because of pain on a treadmill that went 1 ½ mph. After the 5-month period was over those on the regular American diet were able to walk 3 times as far. That's good. That's what the average man can do without changing his diet. But those on our diet were able to walk 50 times as far. It's an absolute record. There's nowhere in the world where this has been approached. Diet and exercise are going to give you a tremendous amount of capability. Whereas you try and do it with exercise alone your just not going to make it. Today you go to a vascular surgeon they pull out the old roto rooter and clear out your main arteries but you have 60,000 miles in your artery tree, they have not figured out how to drill out the vessels in the brain, or eyes.

The Tarahumara Indians of Northern Mexico eat no refined foods. It's identical to the diet I recommend: corn, peas, squash, native fruit and vegetables. They have a small amount of animal protein a few times a month. The Tarahumara are the blood relatives of the Pima Indians in our country. They split off about 400 years a go. The Pima's eat the American kind of diet and eat more of it then most Americans they eat probably 2000 calories of fat a day. The Pima's have more heart disease, arthritis, diabetes, gallstones than any group in the country. While the Tarahumara have none of these diseases-- heart disease is unknown. If you are a runner you know the Tarahumara. The Tahahumara have a kickball game where they run 150 miles continuously day and night for 48 hours. That's real endurance.

A Dr. Bassler erroneous theory: If you didn't smoke and you can run a marathon in less than 4 hours, you would be immune from a heart attack immune from atherosclerosis. That was thrown out when this report was published by B. F. Waller and W. C. Roberts, pathologists at the National Institute of Health. Their conclusion was coronary heart disease appears to be the major killer of conditioned runners aged 40 years and over who die while running.

Jim Shettler's sudden death shocked the running community. Jim had trained like a marathoner since the age of 15. Lean at 6 feet 1 inch and 150 pounds, he had a slow pulse and low blood pressure. He was a nonsmoker and had competed for 25 years in 3000-meter to 10- mile runs. He had run many marathons. On a day in 1976, at age 42, he ran for 3 hours over hilly terrain in preparation for his next marathon. The following day, in Oakland, California, he died.

The autopsy was very clear: a main left artery was almost entirely closed with cholesterol deposits. There was little question that this blockage had created a fatal arrhythmia (irregular heartbeat) and sudden death.

Pritikin advised people who eat SAD not to run or even play singles tennis. People who do aerobic exercise have 50% less upper respiratory infections and recover in half the time vs people who don't.

While running is an aerobic sport of endurance, intended to really get your blood pumping, weightlifting is a feat of strength. It has a different effect on your heart, too. Contracting all of these large muscle groups dramatically increases blood pressure over a very short period of time. The heart responds by getting bigger and thicker—but the growth happens in the heart muscle itself, not in the chambers, the heart-pumping cardiovascular drama of endurance exercise may seem sufficient, but that's not the case. Strength training is among the most important things for people to do after age 50 for building and maintaining strong bones and muscles in an entirely different realm from walking or running or biking. People think you don't need to lift weights because you run, that's not true. Researches have proved strength training is more effective at weight loss then aerobic exercise.

HIIT High Intensity Interval training improves insulin resistance, 15 minutes you can burn 350 calories. Tabata is the name of the Japanese researcher who discovered HIIT you can download an app for your smartphone which has a simple HIIT program called Tabata. HIIT may be better than all other exercises for heart health and improving aerobic capacity and fitness. Check out www.ntnu.edu/cerg

Fitness should be as recreational as possible participating with friends, family or classes makes it more social and enjoyable but just don't rely on any of them it's your health. A week of exercise should have cardiovascular, resistance training, HIIT, dynamic stretching, yoga meditation or mindfulness. You may have to create the time.

When I tried to persuade my friends to join my gym the standard excuse was I don't have the time. I would give my standard reply "Excuses are the crutches of the weak". But now I tell them I don't have time not to work out"

Pritikin to demonstrate his diet and exercise philosophy sponsored 6 individuals (who followed the Pritikin program) in the Hawaiian ironman (2 ½ mile ocean swim,100mile bike race and then run a marathon. They finished 1st, 2nd, 3rd, and 4th amazing. Dr. Fuhrman has several world class athletes he councils one a 38 year old, police officer in St. Louis who bench presses 580 lbs.

FOOD IS MEDICINE

The whole food plant based diet for reversing diabetes, preventing heart disease, reducing your risk of cancer, depression, dementia and obtaining a healthy weight

- 2 servings of beans

- ½ cup of berries

- 2 servings of cruciferous vegetables at least one raw

- 2 large salads, one with lunch and one with dinner

- 1 pound of Greens the more greens you eat the more weights you lose

- 1 or 2 servings of bean vegetable soup. preferable homemade

- 2 servings of other vegetables

- 4 serving of fruits

- Flaxseed 1 or 2 table spoons and a vitaminB 12 200mg supplement prevent heart attacks in vegans

- 1 to 3 Oz of nuts

- Spices one teaspoon of turmeric and one teaspoon of amla (Indian gooseberry)

- Seeds (Chia best for diabetics) sunflower sesame, pumpkin

- Herbs all kinds

- 3 servings of whole grains

- Torfu

- Beverages healthiest water, coffee, tea, soy and or almond milk one oz of pomegranate juice

- Exercise 1 hour a day everyday

- Sweeteners: Stevia, Date sugar, Erythritol

- Stevia should be limited to 1.8 mg per pound of body weight

- Smoothie lots of frozen berries and organic greens almond or soy milk easy

- Salad Dressing should ideally be nut and fruit based lots of receipts on the internet

- Healthy salad dressing is a key without oil or animal products

You need a powerful blender like a Vitamix for salad dressings smoothies, and Sorbet

You should know all your health numbers, check your vitamin D3 level most Americans are deficient your mineral levels and your EPA DHA

SUGGESTIONS

Breakfast

- ½ cup of steel cut oats or 1 cup for men

- ½ cup of berries, table spoon flaxseed meal 1 teaspoon turmeric

- 6 walnut halves and a low sugar fruit

- 1 oz of pomegranate juice

Lunch

- Big salad

- One serving of any type of fruit is ok because the sugar load will be diluted with the rest of the vegetable

- Vegetable bean soup

- Steamed or cooked greens

Dinner

- Another salad

- Large plate of steamed green vegetables

- Raw vegetables with dip: tomato based salsa-type or hummus

- Cup of beans

- Fruit salad

GREAT SUPPORT

Nathan Pritikin commented in one of his lectures that he had alumni from his health spa diabetic for 20 years on 80 units of insulin get off all their insulin in 6 weeks and have better blood sugar. Mr. Pritikin is no longer with us but his Health Spa is, if you have 6 thousand dollars you wish to spend. I suggest people who are on medication and need support become a member of Dr. Joel Fuhrman's website www.drfuhrman.com. Dr. Fuhrman has helped thousands of patients become non-diabetic and reversed other chronic diseases. You should read the testimonials. Dr. Fuhrman also has gourmet chiefs creating wonderful receipts making your journey to health more enjoyable. His patient forum allows people to share their successes, recipes and support for people experiencing similar diseases.

How does this work?

Most diabetics lose 100 pounds the first year assuming they need to lose that much weight you start pulling out the fat and toxins from your organs and tissue and replacing with all those protective micronutrients. When you eat greens, blueberries, strawberries your pee doesn't turn green, blue or red these stay in your body healing and protecting. When you stop insulting your body 3 or 4 times a day with toxic food your body heals remember Dr. Gregor's best keep secret in medicine given the right circumstance the body will heal itself.

Natural Forces within us are the true healers of disease. Hippocrates

No snacking especially after dinner your healing your pancreas and it's exhausted beta cells fasting from dinner to breakfast is a good thing

ORGANIC FOOD THE "DIRTY DOZEN"

12 Most Contaminated	12 Least Contaminated

Peaches	Onions
Apples	Avocado
Sweet bell peppers	Sweet Corn (Frozen)
Nectarines	Pineapples
Strawberries	Mango
Cherries	Asparagus
Pears	Sweet Peas (Frozen)
Grapes (imported)	Kiwi Fruit
Spinach	Bananas
Lettuce	Cabbage
Potatoes	Broccoli
Celery	Papaya

HELPFUL SUGGESTIONS

- Plan your meals the previous evening for the next day

- Keep a pot of beans in the fridge for bean burritos, throw on salads, bean dip, humus or just a plane bowel of beans

- Greens use in smoothies, add to vegetable bean soup, on salads, steamed, water sautéed

- Cook lightly add a pepper sauce or a balsamic vinaigrette

- Good Investment Instant pot cooker on Amazon Smart Bluetooth-enabled multifunction pressure cooker lots of vegan cookbooks for the Instant Pot. So you can run on your treadmill and cook dinner at the same time

- Healthy Bread Ezekiel 4.9 Dave's Bread the thin sliced

- Drink lots of water

- Keep toxic food out of your home

- Frozen vegetables and fruit is often better picked frozen same day no ppreservatives

Meals can be as exotic or as simple as you chose going vegan does not mean a bland and boring diet I've found it more enjoyable and it didn't take me long 6 to 8weeks and I grew up on a family cattle ranch with a walk in meat freezer

Dr. Furhman allows 8 to 10 oz of wild fish or range free skinless chicken a week no red meat or processed meat optional as a condiment. He also adds this may prevent some people from achieving their goals.

Moderate changes in diet can leave one with moderate blindness, moderate kidney failure, and moderate amputations.

Dr. Dean Ornish noted that "the Mediterranean diet had no significant reduction in the rates of heart attack, death from cardiovascular causes, or death from any cause," but it reduced stroke risk by 50%. The authors of the study replied that may be true, but the major problem with Ornish's diet is that it doesn't taste good, and so, hardly anyone sticks to it.

But it's not true. Ornish got extraordinary adherence in his studies with no difference in any of the acceptability measures; same enjoyment compared to their regular diet. They even got success in barbecue country, rural North Carolina. See, stricter diets may meet greater acceptance among patients than more modest diets because they may work better. Greater adherence means greater disease reversal.

But you don't have to be facing certain death. Even those who are young and healthy with no health problems had no problem sticking to a plant based diet. In fact, it worked a little too well. This was a crossover study where they asked people to eat plant-based for a few months and then switch back to their baseline diet to note the contrast, but people felt so good eating healthy some refused to go back to their regular diet, which kind of messes up the study. They were losing weight with no calorie counting or portion control, they had more energy, their periods got better, better digestion, better sleep-many were like no way, we're not going back.

Pay Attention: The study that purported to show that diets high in meat, eggs, and dairy could be as harmful to health as smoking supposedly suggested that people under 65 who eat lots of meat, eggs, and dairy are four times as likely to die from cancer or diabetes. But if you look at the actual study, you'll see that's not true. Those eating a lot of animal protein didn't have just four times more risk of dying from diabetes, they had 73 times higher risk of dying from diabetes. (Sample,1 2014 Diets high in meat, eggs and dairy)

For maximizing weight loss, the trick is to use beans as your primary starch source and only one other serving a day of a non-beans starchy food like beets, carrots, peas, and squashes. If you're eating a one-cup serving of a starch whole grain, such as oatmeal, steel-cut oats, or wild rice with breakfast, do not eat the starch vegetable option with dinner.

High-starch foods made from flour, rice, or white potatoes should be eliminated from your diet; no fruit drinks, eat the fruit instead, no sodas, no trans fat, keep saturated fat below 10%.

Raw vegetables and all cooked green and non-starch vegetables; string beans, artichokes, zucchini, snow peas, eggplant, tomatoes, peppers, mushrooms, cauliflower, onions, and leeks. You do not have to measure-- eat as much as you like remember two cups of beans a day.

While most of the common carbohydrates we eat are turned into glucose. the conversion efficiency and rate vary greatly from one type of carbohydrate to another. The starch in potatoes, cereals, and baked goods digests very rapidly and all their calories are converted quickly, supplying the body with a hug glucose load. The starch in beans, barley, and black wild rice is digested more slowly and causes a much slower and lower blood sugar rise. Unique properties of the carbohydrate in beans and legumes are higher amount of slowly digestible starch, resistant starch, insoluble fiber, and higher amount of soluble fiber. Resistant starch is the secret. There are different types of resistant starch in foods. Amylose and amylopectin are examples. It is starch that is tightly packed in a stable crystalline form within foods, making it difficult to digest. The more resistant starch that reaches the colon undigested, the less calories we absorb from that food. When resistant starch reaches the colon, the bacteria there use it for fuel. The resistant starch is also, therefore, a prebiotic, meaning it serves to fuel the growth of beneficial bacteria in the colon.

Degrading these starches by bacterial action is called fermentation, and it produces a type of fat called short-chain fatty acids(SCFAs). In other words, the resistant starch does not even get converted to a simple sugar; it gets converted into a simple fat. Only a small percent of these calories are absorbed by the body, but are highly beneficial. So calories from resistant starch are listed on the food labels but almost 90 percent of those calories do not get absorbed and they do not raise blood sugar at all. Resistant starch is especially associated with one type of SCFA called butyrate.

Now here's the fascinating part: even though only a small amount gets absorbed, butyrate offers a wide array of health benefits, including strong protection against colon cancer. It protects our bodies in lots of other ways too, namely by enhancing the absorption of beneficial minerals like calcium and magnesium and so, importantly, improving insulin sensitivity. It has the opposite effect of eating sugary or high glycemic starches. It actually improves diabetic glucose numbers the day after it's eaten.

Most importantly, these SCFAs slow down glycolysis in the liver, thus delaying hunger, and they increase the breakdown of body fat as a source of energy, facilitating weight loss. Glycolysis is the breakdown of the stored glycogen back into glucose for use by the body. The small amount of SCFAS that are absorbed increases fat oxidation, meaning your body burns fat for energy more efficiently, encouraging weight loss.

When you eat a meal of mostly green vegetables, eggplant, onions, mushrooms, and a cup of beans, biochemical events occur that work medicinally; they repair the biochemical defects that lead to diabetes.

Second meal effect the remarkable effect of beans to help control blood sugar not just the meal your having with beans but hours later or even the next day. The good bacteria feed by the beans manufacture compounds like propronate which gets absorbed into our system and slows down the gastric emptying, slows the rate at which food leaves our stomach so we don't get as much of a sugar rush. Second meal is not correct description more like 3 or 4 meal affects and the benefits continue as long as you consume beans.

Bean consumption has been associated with lower body weight, waist circumference, risk of overweight or obesity and systolic blood pressure in epidemiological studies.

Whether the association of bean consumption with healthier body weight and risk factors of the metabolic syndrome is due to physiological effects of pulses or simply an indicator of a healthy lifestyle is uncertain. You know if a person is smart enough to eat beans maybe they are eating all kinds of healthy foods and exercise. So, researchers wanted to know; reduction in waist circumference should be a primary goal of strategies designed to reduce risk factors associated with the metabolic syndrome and reducing the risk of prediabetes turning into full blown diabetes.

Energy restriction is the cornerstone of most weight-loss strategies however, evidence suggests that the majority of individuals who lose weight regain it during subsequent months or years. Starving yourself seldom works, thus it is important to identify foods that can be easily incorporated into the diet and spontaneously lead to the attainment and maintenance of a healthy body weight and improved metabolic control. The test compared frequent pulse consumption as a dietary intervention in an ad libitum diet (diet didn't change) and caloric restriction group with dietary counselling to reduce energy intake on risk factors of the metabolic syndrome in overweight and obese adults.

The bean group was asked to eat five cups a week of lentils, chickpeas, yellow split peas and navy beans. So, the bean group was asked to eat more food. The 5 cups were added to their regular diet.

The cutting calorie group was asked to eat less food and the more food group won not only was regularly consuming pulses as effective at reducing risk factors as an energy restricted. Both diets led to reduced energy intakes and waist circumference, improved glycemic control and insulin sensitivity, the pulse diet, had additional benefits, perhaps due to some functional properties of pulses. The researchers concluded frequent consumption of pulses in an ad libitum diet reduced risk factors of the Metabolic syndrome and these were, equivalent in some instances stronger, than counselling for dietary energy reduction of 500 calories a day.

Don't use Beano as it reduces the restricted starch. Chew your beans well and it leads to less gas and your body will adjust. You might start out with smaller portion sizes.

BEANS

Health authorities from all over the world universally recommend increasing the consumption of whole grains and legumes for health promoting diets. And one of the reasons is that they may decrease insulin resistance, the defining trait of type 2 diabetes.

Pay Attention: OHAs and insulin are the mainstay of the treatment of diabetes and are effective in controlling hyperglycemia. They have prominent side effects and fail to significantly alter the course of diabetic complications. Common side effects include weight gain, swelling, liver disease. Let me repeat! The mainstay of diabetic treatment fails to significantly alter the course of diabetic complications. Shouldn't that be the whole point of treatment?

Thankfully, lifestyle modifications have proven to be greatly effective in the management of this disease, and if there is one thing diabetics should eat, it's legumes: beans, chickpeas, split peas, and lentils.

The European Association for the Study of Diabetes, the Canadian Diabetes Association, and the American Diabetes Association all recommend the consumption of dietary pulses as a means of optimizing diabetes control. What are pulses? They're peas and beans that come dried, so a subset of legumes, so excluding green beans and fresh green peas also the so-called oilseeds: soybeans and peanuts.

Chickpeas got high marks and in terms of beans, while pintos and black beans may beat out kidney beans. Compared to the blood sugar spike of straight white rice, black beans and rice, and pinto beans and rice appeared to beat out kidney beans and rice. This may be because dark red kidney beans can have lower levels of indigestible starch. One of the reason beans are so healthy is they contain compounds that partially block our starch digesting enzyme, which allows some starch to make it down to our colon to feed our good gut bacteria. In fact, the inhibition of this starch-eating enzyme, amylase, just by eating beans, approximates that of a carb-blocking drug, acarbose, sold as precise, a popular diabetes medication. The long-term use of beans may normalize hemoglobin A1C levels (which is how you track diabetes) almost as well as the drug, without drug side effects. (Dr. Fuhrman's Immunity Solution! 2015)

SALAD VEGETABLES

- Lettuces all varieties

- Tomatoes

- Carrots Radishes

- Fennel

- String Beans

- English Peas

- Hearts of Palm

- Celery

- Broccoli

- Cauliflower Baby Bok Choy

- Snap Peas

- Endive,

- Water Chestnuts

- Zucchini

- Onions and Scallions

- Sprouts

- Cucumber

- Snow Peas

- Peppers

- Stewed Mushrooms (chilled) Mushrooms are best cooked, even stewed, for a few minutes. They contain a mild toxin called agaritine, that dissipates with even light cooking. Mushrooms have powerful anticancer effects, and those powers are likely enhanced by cooking them.

THE WORLD'S HEALTHIEST FOOD: CRUCIFEROUS VEGETABLES

- Kale
- Collards
- Broccoli
- Broccoli Rabe
- Brocollina
- Brussels sprouts
- Watercress
- Bok Choy
- Cabbage
- Chinese Cabbage
- Mustard Greens
- Arugula
- Kohlrabi
- Red Cabbage
- Mache
- Turnip Greens
- Horseradish
- Rutabaga

- Turnips

- Radishes

- Cauliflower

While eating fresh fruits, beans, vegetables, seeds and nuts has been shown in scientific studies to reduce the occurrence of cancer, cruciferous vegetables are different. Instead it has a one-to-two relationship with a wide variety of human cancers. In other words, as plant food intake goes up 20 percent in a population, cancer rates typically drop 20 percent. But as cruciferous vegetable intake goes up 20 percent, cancer rates typically drop 40 percent.

- Detoxify toxins and carcinogens, rendering them harmless

- Regulate the liver's ability to remove toxins

- Remove free radicals to prevent oxidative and DNA damage in cells

- Transform hormones into beneficial compounds that inhibit hormone-sensitive cancers

- Enhance and protect against age related loss of cellular glutathione

- Enable cell death in cells that have abnormal mutations and DNA damage

- Maximizing the benefits of Cruciferous Vegetables

Methods of preparation and cooking affect the availability of ITC's to be digested and absorbed. Chopping, chewing, blending, and juicing all allow for enhanced production of ITC's. In other words, these beneficial ITC's are not preformed in the plant; they are made in our mouth from glucosinolate precursors as we chew and crush the cell walls. The more cell walls that are broken, the more myrosinase (an enzyme housed in the cell membrane) that is released and can be mixed with the glucosinolates inside the cell to catalyze the reaction that makes ITCs.

Some ITC benefit may be lost with boiling or steaming, as myrosinase enzyme can be destroyed with too much heat; so the maximum benefit from eating cruciferous vegetables raw. However, some production of ITC in cooked cruciferous vegetables may still occur, because the bacteria in the digestive tract have some myrosinase activity. The myrosinase-producing ability of gut bacteria can be increased with regular consumption of green vegetables.

Keep in mind that cooking does not destroy the activity and function of the ITCs; it only deactivates the enzyme catalyzing their formation. That means if you blend, crush, chop, or juice the greens while they're raw to maximize the ITC production and then put the blended or chopped greens into a stew or soup to cook, you will still have those functioning and beneficial ITCs present after cooking. Chew all cruciferous greens very, very, well. Puree, blend, or chop cruciferous vegetables before adding them to stews or soups.

Natural forces within us are the true healers of disease Hippocrates The hundred plus ITCs found in cruciferous vegetables enhance our own immune system greatly. I can't emphasize the importance of the health benefits from cruciferous vegetables enough.

GREENS AND HEART DISEASE

Heart disease is caused by the buildup of fatty plaques in the arteries, known as atherosclerosis. However, arteries do not get clogged up with these plaques in a uniform way. Bends and branches of blood vessels-where blood flow is disrupted and can be sluggish-are much more prone to the buildup. A recent study shows that Nrf2, a protein that usually protects against plaque buildup, is inactive in areas of arteries that are prone to disease. However, a phytochemical found in green vegetables activates Nrf2 in these disease-prone regions. Activation of Nrf2 is important for maximizing both prevention and removal of plaque. Ingestion of these beneficial compounds from cruciferous green vegetables had the strongest effect to activate the Nrf2 proteins, blocking atherosclerosis.

WHOLE GRAINS

An analysis of a bunch of randomized drug trials suggests that taking a blood pressure lowering medication for high blood pressure may reduce the risk of getting a heart attack by 15%, and the risk of getting a stoke by about 25%. What a coincidence. A recent study found that we may achieve similar benefits eating just three portions of whole grains a day. The observed decrease in systolic blood pressure could decrease the incidence of coronary artery disease and stroke by 15% and 25%, respectively'.

While whole grains are good, refined grains may not just be neutral.

Out of Harvard- "White Rice, Brown Rice, and Risk of Type 2 Diabetes".

In these three prospective cohort studies of US men and women, they found that regular consumption of white rice was associated with higher risk of type 2 diabetes, whereas brown rice intake was associated with lower risk. An interesting wrinkle is that they found other whole grains may be even better than brown rice.

Eating white rice was associated with a 17% greater risk of diabetes. Replace with brown, and instead apparently get a 16% drop in risk. And replace white rice with other whole grains, such as oats and barley—a 36% lower diabetes risk. Just a single serving a day of oats and barley may lower our cholesterol. Whole grains are more than just refined grains with a fiber coat. With white flour, you just get the bran but all the rest of nutrition is stripped away which includes most of the compounds responsible for whole grain contributions to the health of our bowels, with, blood sugar, cancer prevention, bones, brain and heart.

FLAXSEED

A daily tablespoon of ground flaxseed for a month appears to improve fasting blood sugars, triglycerides, cholesterol, and hemoglobin A1C levels in diabetics. World Health Organization researchers published an open-label study on the effect of flax seed powder in the management of diabetes. Flaxseed may improve insulin sensitivity in glucose intolerant people. Not recommend flaxseed supplementation during pregnancy. You can buy the seed in bulk and then grind with a coffee grinder or buy the meal.

PROCESSED FOOD A GREAT DAMAGE

If someone wishes for good health one must first ask oneself if he is ready to do away with the reasons for his illness. Only then is it possible to help him. Hippocrates

The Standard American Diet (SAD) is 54% processed food 32% meat products only about 10% is fruit and vegetables and most of that is white potatoes which we consume as processed food French fries or potato chips and 4% whole grains. (Dr. Joel Fuhrman's Immunity Solution! 2015)

To have a healthy life you have to have a healthy weight 80% of Americans are overweight the longest living people have a bmi below 23 most Americans have a bmi above 25.

When you process food you remove the beneficial compounds, fiber, and antioxidants you just get the calories, empty calories. The more processed foods you put in your body the more your aging and setting up yourself for chronic diseases and cancer.

Food is made up of Macronutrients: proteins, carbohydrates and fat all contain calories also water but it doesn't contain calories. Food also is made up of Micronutrients vitamins, minerals and phytochemical which contain no calories.

Excesses of Macronutrients damages our bodies causes weight gain and degenerative diseases. Your health and longevity depends on the consumption of Micronutrients.

Cancer fighting food are also fat storage fighting foods preventing new blood vessels developing to feed the fat understand fat is like a tumor it needs new blood vessels to grow.

Your diet should be Hormonal favorable. Foods with high Glycemic loads like white flour which is not much different than refined sugar causes an insulin spike because it's quickly digested and released into the blood stream and the body can't use it as energy so it's stored as fat insulin promotes fat storage.

Meat products promote the growth hormone IGF 1 (Insulin Growth Factor One) is associated with every step in the development of cancer. Along with promoting fat storage.

In a study of 6000,50-65 years old men and women over 18 years those eating 20% of their diet in meat protein had a 4 fold increase risk of cancer and a 75% increased risk of death. Another study over 22 years they gave the participants a value of 1 to 20 those eating the least animal protein got a 1 those eating the most got a value of 20. The ones who had a value of 16-20 had 60 times increase risk of cardiac death.

Food addiction calories absorb fast signals dopamine receptors in the brain it only last a few seconds but it keeps you thinking, without proper nutrients you acquire perverted cravings.

Your stomach only holds a liter so the term crowding out replacing dangerous food with high nutrient food which trigger nutrient receptors resulting in less appetite. A pound of raw vegetables is less than 100 calories.

Detoxification withdrawal you will feel worse from detoxification you have to feel worse to get better. It doesn't last long a few days a week maybe.

Your body has two phases in regards to food Anabolic absorption phase (eating) and the catabolic phase burn off phase. Americans spend very little time in the catabolic phase usually when they are sleeping. Spending more time living in the catabolic phase means you get to spend more time living.

The body has two types of fat subcutaneous fat the fat you can squeeze like your love handles the other visceral fat is deeper mixed in and around your organs, the dangerous fat. When you yo yo diet you gain the fat back again (scientific studies suggest around 90% gain the weight back) but it comes back as visceral fat increasing your risk of diabetes heart disease think of Tom Hanks often losing weight for acting roles it caught up with him now he has type 2 diabetes. He mentioned his doctor told him he would have to lose down to his high school weight to become non-diabetic and he said he weight 90 lbs. in high school so that was not going to happen. Who knows if that is true or not but all he has to do is lose down to his healthy weight and most people reverse their diabetes in a few months. Look at the study from open access, If Hanks doctor did tell him that he needs to get a different doctor or go back to his character Forrest Gump he liked to run and eat a high nutrient diet.

Americans eat around 400 calories of oil a day oil is a fast food enters the blood stream fast the body hates fat in its blood stream so it stores it, from your lips to your hips less than 15 minutes, oil is a processed food.

You need to look at this as an adventure a new experience but it's a new lifestyle that can prevent you from experiencing the chronic diseases everyone who eats the SAD will sooner or later succumb. The Standard American Diet is a serial killer You're not unique really it's that simple.

Pritikin said you can retrain your palate in 30 days and lose your taste for salt in as little as a week but the emotional attachment may last as long as a year. Pritikin longevity center has almost a

90% compliance. I know you can't achieve this by shear will and accepting deprivation not going to happen because the primitive part of your brain is saying you can't do this, they have lots of medicine, you're just a little over weight it happens with age you under too much stress too take on something like changing your lifestyle and the loss of pleasure of eating all those unhealthy meals. You see that voice inside your head is a liar. The unhealthy meals are giving you stress after a period of time you will enjoy healthy food more than the toxic food. I lost 22 pounds in about 6 weeks but I could have lost 200 pounds I'm still eating a high nutrient diet after 2 years. I'm just at my healthy weight. People lose an average of 13 pounds a month. Another thing I've noticed I need less calories for stamina my body is more efficient with the food. This is not a diet it's a healthy way of life.

The first duck season with this lifestyle. I showed up at the duck club with my salad, vegetable bean soup, oatmeal, and fruit great bunch of guys well except one, there is always a horse's ass, nevertheless I expected the kidding it's no big deal (my brother had just had open heart surgery a few weeks before duck season). After a while Drew the asshole says just like you Moore going to extremes it was his tone. You know Drew getting cut almost in half that's extreme, eating a bean burrito walk in the park. The following weekend Randy and I are on the front porch of the club it's around 5am just enjoying the stillness and Drew drives up in his new jeep with his undisciplined lab named Drake. Drew gets out and closes the door, leaving the jeep running. Drake jumps into the driver's seat and starts pawing the window and hits the automatic door lock. The German word is Schadenfreude pleasure taken at the misfortunes of someone else. Drew first tried to coach Drake to hit the automatic door lock not going to happen. I offered to break out a window least I could do. Enough Schadenfreude I gave Drew my cellphone and keys to my truck suggested he call his wife meet her half way get the keys and still get back for the morning hunt. As he walked to my truck, Randy assured Drew we would watch Drake and make sure he didn't drive off. He flipped us the bird and smiled as he got in the truck.

Threshold no one knows how much meat or processed food is acceptable but we do know from the Adventist study and epidemiology studies, intervention studies, prospective studies the more plant based are diets the healthier our species.

Big Food have PHDs combining fat, sugar, salt and oil to see what is most additive checking how the brain reacts with high tech instruments. I'm all about personal responsibility but this is predatory and the government should stop it.

Permission slip that's what one famous life style doctor called a prescription instead of counseling their patient to lose weight and eat a healthy diet and exercise. That's the problem with the American Health Industry they are not reimbursed for counseling and most have no nutritional training.

The day I finished this attempt to help an article in my local paper announced the life expectancy had declined in the United States December 12, 2016.

Dairy, growing research points to bovine insulin as a possible cause of Type one diabetes. Infants fed milk or formula and from their Mother who drinks milk. Childhood cancers; the Mothers not only have to be concerned about what they eat while their pregnant but before, women who eat lots of green leafy vegetables 2 years before pregnancy and during pregnancy have children with less childhood cancers. Vitamin A and folic acid should not be taken, folic acid recommended for pregnant women is been shown to cause and increase risk of breast cancer and is also detrimental to the child causing an increased risk of allergies. You need folate from leafy greens, fresh fruits, and legumes. Not a pill! (Dr. Fuhrman immunity solution 2015)

When someone suggest to you a diet the first thing you should ask does this prevent the number one killer in the western world heart disease. The same diet that protects against heart disease protects against diabetes, cancer and Alzheimer's it's the same diet.

One of the most remarkable documented demonstration of the power of plants I've read was Dr. Joe Crowe who later replaced Dr. Caldwell Esselstyn as head of the Breast Institute at the Cleveland Clinic. After Dr. Crowe's heart attack in 1996 test showed that the entire left anterior descending coronary artery-the vessels leading to the front of the heart and nicknamed "the widow-maker"- was significantly diseased. His coronary artery anatomy excluded him as a candidate for surgical bypass, angioplasty, or stents, and at such a young age with a wife and three small children.

Dr. Esselstyn invited Dr. Crowe and his wife to his home for dinner. This gave Dr. Esselstyn time to explain his research. Both Dr. Crowe and his wife immediately grasped the implications for Joe of a plant based diet. Dr. Esselstyn said he redefined the word commitment. He stuck to the plan rigorously, eventually reducing his total blood cholesterol count to just 89/dL and cutting his LDL, or "bad" cholesterol, from 98 mg/dL to 38 mg/dL.

After two and a half years after Joe adopted a strict plant-based diet, there came a point when he was exceptionally busy professionally, under considerable stress. And he noted a return of some discomfort in his chest. His cardiologists asked for more test.

On the day of his follow-up angiogram Dr. Esselstyn went by his office and when they greeted he notice moisture in Dr. Crowe's eye and asked "Is everything OK?"

"You saved my life". He declared, "It's gone! It's not there anymore! Something lethal is gone! My follow-up angiogram was normal."

Dr. Esselstyn asked Dr. Crowe years later what made him decide to change, he responded very simply. "We believed you", and added I had nothing else. (Prevent and Reverse Heart Disease Caldwell B. Esselstyn, Jr., M.D.)

Dr. Esselstyn won a gold medal in the 1956 Olympic Games as the number six oar on the victorious US rowing team and 1968 was awarded the Bronze star in Vietnam as an Army surgeon

"Nobody can go back and start a New beginning, but anyone can start today and make a new Ending" (Maria Robinson)

NOTES, REFERENCES AND LIST

Angiogenesis inhibition: prevents tumors from growing, prevents fat cells from expanding, prevents inflammation, inhibits development of cancer.

- Allium vegetables (onion family)

- Berries (all types)

- Black rice

- Cinnamon

- Citrus fruit

- Cruciferous vegetables

- Flax seeds

- Ginger

- Grapes

- Green Tea

- Mushrooms

- Omega-3 fats

- Peppers

- Pomegranate

- Quince

- Resveratrol (from grapes and red wine

- Soybeans

- Spinach

- Tomatoes

- Turmeric

These foods are listed in alphabetical order, not in the order of their angiogenesis-inhibiting effects.

RESISTANT STARCH + FIBER IN COMMON PLANT FOODS

Food	%RS	%Fiber	%RS + Fiber
Black Beans	26.9	42.6	69.5
Northern Beans	28.0	41.1	69.1
Navy beans	25.9	36.2	62.1
Red Kidney beans	24.6	36.8	61.4
Lentils	25.4	33.1	58.5
Split peas	24.5	33.1	57.6
Black-eyed peas	17.7	32.6	50.3
Corn	25.2	19.6	44.7
Barley	18.2	17.0	35.2

Brown Rice	14.8	5.1	20.5
Millet	12.6	5.4	18.0
Rolled oats	7.2	10.0	17.2
White Rice	14.1	1.5	15.6
Whole wheat	1.7	12.1	13.8
White Pasta	3.3	5.6	8.9
Sweet Potato		3.0	

UNACCEPTABLE CARBOHYDRATES

All of the above acceptable carbs are rendered unacceptable with excessive processing. In addition, you want to avoid the following:

- Sweeteners, sugar, honey, maple syrup

- White flour

- White rice

- Whole-grain pastry flour

- Packaged cold cereals

- Commercial fruit juices and even fruit-juice-sweetened beverages

High-glycemic, nutrient-sparse processed foods are not just fattening, they also suppress the immune system and increase the risk of cancer. Most of us are unaware that croissants, white bread, bagels, pasta, cakes, cupcakes, pancakes, and most other "white" foods have been linked to many different types of cancer. "The whiter your bread the sooner you're dead." "The more you eat green the more you get lean." (Dr. Joel Fuhrman author of Eat to Live)

UNDERSTANDING THE GLYCEMIC INDEX

Studies evaluating the negative effects of a higher glycemic diet revealed that foods composed of low-nutrient, low-fiber, processed grains and sweets have deficiencies, and they harm far beyond their glycemic response. Processed foods are also low in fiber, phytonutrients and antioxidants and are rich in toxic acrylamides. In addition to having a high GL, they are disease promoting foods. When a diet is rich in nutrients the disease-protective qualities of these foods and their weight-loss benefits overwhelm any insignificant drawback from their moderate GL.

Food	Glycemic Index	Glycemic Load
White Potato (1 medium baked)	90	29
White Rice (1 cup cooked)	68	29
Brown Rice	58	24
White Pasta	53	21
Chocolate Cake (1/10 box cake mix +2T frosting)	38	20
Raisins (1/4 cup)	64	19
Corn (1cup cooked)	52	18
Sweet Potato (1 medium baked)	69	14
Black rice (1 cup)	65	14
Grapes (1 cup)	59	14
Rolled Oats (1 cup)	55	13

Whole wheat (1cup cooked)	30	11
Mango (1 cup)	51	11
Lentils (1 cup cooked)	40	9
Apple (1 medium)	39	9
Kiwi (2 medium)	58	8
Green Peas (1 cup cooked)	53	8
Butternut Squash (1 cup cooked)	51	8
Kidney Beans (1 cup cooked)	22	7
Blueberries (1 cup)	53	7
Black Beans (1 cup cooked)	20	6
Watermelon (1 cup)	76	6
Orange (1 medium)	37	4
Cashews (1 ounce)	25	2
Carrots (1 cup cooked)	39	3
Carrots (1 cup raw)	35	2
Strawberries (1 cup)	10	1
Cauliflower	negligible	negligible
Eggplant	negligible	negligible
Tomatoes	negligible	negligible
Mushrooms	negligible	negligible
Onions	negligible	negligible

FOODS THAT ARE HARMFUL FOR HEALTH

Diabetics mostly die of heart attacks. A meat-based diet promotes atherosclerosis, increases the risk of blood clots, and accelerates kidney failure in diabetics. A diet high in animal products and low in vegetables and beans is the formula for a medical disaster. Diabetics need the opposite: a diet high in vegetables and beans and low in animal products.

Some people have bought into the faulty logic that if sugar and refined grains and other high-glycemic foods raise blood sugar and triglycerides, then we should eat more animal products instead. Unquestionably, sugar, white flour, and other processed grains are unfavorable and must be removed to achieve good health, but to increase animal products at the expense of vegetables, beans, nuts and seeds, and over low-glycemic, nutrient-rich plant foods (which are protein adequate) is not only dangerous but also reduces the potential for the diabetic to recover and get off all medications.

The main problem with recommending a diet with a significant amount of animal products for diabetics is that the increased protein intake promotes the progression of diabetic kidney disease, and the animal-source protein and saturated fat intake raise cholesterol and promote heart disease. Even though a protein-dense diet might offer some marginal weight loss benefits compared to a diet with lots of processed carbohydrates, it still does not allow the substantive weight reduction that diabetics really need to rid themselves of the disease.

Emerging evidence also suggests that carbohydrate-restrictive, also called ketogenic, diets create metabolic derangement conducive to cardiac conduction abnormalities and/or myocardial dysfunction. In other words, it may cause other potentially life-threatening heart problems. Ketogenic diets are the most dangerous. Medical literature has shown them to cause cardiomyopathy, a pathological enlargement of the heart that is reversible but only if the diet is stopped in time. Even following a ketogenic diet short term, such as with the induction phase of the Atkins or Dukan diets, is dangerous, and deaths have occurred from cardiac arrhythmias induced from the electrolyte derangement.

A landmark study published in 2000 actually measured what was happening to the arteries of people on low-carb, high-protein diets. Utilizing SPECT scans to directly measure blood flow within coronary arteries, the development of heart disease was examined in sixteen people on a vegetarian diet that was high in fruits and vegetables and in ten people on a low-carb, high-animal-protein diet. The results were shocking. Those sticking to the whole foods vegetarian diet showed a reversal in expected heart disease. The partially clogged arteries literally got cleaned out, and blood flow to their heart through their coronary arteries increased by 40 percent. Those on the high-protein diet exhibited rapid advancement of their heart disease with a 40 percent decrease in blood flow in the heart's blood vessels. Thus, the only study on high-protein diet to actually measure arterial blood flow showed that this style of eating is exceedingly dangerous

Red meats are to be avoided completely. Studies on diabetics and meat eating indicate a 50 percent higher incidence of heart disease in people with high red meat intake. Researchers believe this in not associated with the higher levels of saturated fat in red meat but instead with the heme iron it contains. It is increased consumption of both processed foods and animal products that is linked to increased mortality, diabetes, and heart problems. Large-scale studies of the metabolic syndrome have linked the incidence of high glucose, abdominal fat, high triglycerides, and high blood pressure in western societies with red meat, processed meat, fried food, refined grains, and diet soda. When multiple dangerous foods are consumed, it creates a deadly combination.

The metabolic syndrome is a cluster of cardiovascular disease risk factors associated with increased risk of diabetes and mortality. Studies invariably show that the most protection, prevention, and reversal of and lower risk of, heart disease occurs when the diet style is high in vegetables, beans, fruits, and nuts and is very low in animal products.

DISEASES UNCOMMON IN CULTURES WHO EAT A PREDOMINANT WHOLE FOOD PLANT BASED DIET

- Obesity

- Constipation (Americans spend over 80 billion a year treating constipation)

- Arthritis (all three types)

- Gall stones

- Psoriasis (Pritikin said he cured the worst cases in 4 months)

- Glaucoma

- Cataracts

- Diverticulitis (50% of white America over 60 have it, the number is higher with African Americans and at a younger age and most white and black Americans don't know they have it)

- Loss of hearing

- Bowel disorders

- Crohn's disease

- Autoimmune diseases

- Kidney stones

- Heart Disease

- Diabetes

- Colon, prostrate, pancreatic, and breast cancer

- Hypertension

STANDARD AMERICAN DIET

- 60% Refined and Processed food

- 30% Meat Products

- 10% vegetables and fruit primarily white potatoes

And this diet gives us the Standard American Diseases

FAMOUS VEGETARIANS AND VEGANS

- Thomas Edison

- Hippocrates

- Plato

- Leonardo Da Vinci

- Voltaire

- Mary Shelley

- Leo Tolstoy

- Abraham Lincoln

- Albert Einstein (late in life)

- Mohandas Gandhi

- Nikola Tesla

- Clint Eastwood

HELPFUL WEBSITES AND BOOKS

- Nutritionstudies.org. T. Colin Campbell co-author of the China Study great recipes, offers a Plant-based Nutrition Certificate in partnership with eCornell

- Nutritionfacts.org. Michael Greger, md. author of How not to die his Grandmother's life was saved by Nathan Pritikin over 2000 A to Z health videos every health topics

- Drmcdougall.com (Nathan Pritikin was Dr. Mc Dougal's mentor)

- Forkoverknives.com offers a free vegan starter kit

- Plantbasedresearch.org

- cureddiabetes.com Gordon Ritchie

- Bluezone.com offers a questionnaire which estimates your life expectance

- Dr. Dean Ornish lifestyle medicine offers a list of certified Doctors who follow the Ornish Heart disease reversal protocol (heals hearts and transforms lives)

- Dr. David L Katz President of American College of Lifestyle Medicine

- Prevent & Reverse Heart Disease Dr. Esselstyn www.dresselstyn.com

- Eat to Live, The End of Diabetes, Super Immunity by Dr. Joel Fuhrman www.drfuhrman.com

- Dr. Neal Barnard's Program for Reversing Diabetes founding president of the Physicians Committee for Responsible Medicine

- Brain Food Dr. Neal Barnard

- The Alzheimer's Prevention Program Keep your brain healthy Gary Small, MD & Gigi Vorgan

REFERENCES

Agarwal, U., Mishra, S., Xu, J., Levin, S., Gonzales, J., & Barnard, N.D. (2015). A multicenter randomized controlled trial of a nutrition intervention program in a multiethnic adult population in the corporate setting reduces depression and anxiety and improves quality of life: the GEICO study. *Am J Health Promot, 29(4),* 245-254. doi: 10.4278/ajhp.130218-QUAN-72

Blease, C. (2011). Deception as treatment: the case of depression. *J Med Ethics, 37(1),* 13-16. doi:10.1136/jme.2010.039313

Bokulich, N. A., & Blaser, M. J. (2014). A bitter aftertaste: unintended effects of artificial sweeteners on the Gut Microbiome. *Cell Metabolism,* 20(5), 701-703. doi: 10.1016/j.cmet.2014.10.012

Centers for Disease Control and Prevention. (2014). *National Diabetes Statistics Report: Estimates of Diabetes and Its Burden in the United States.* GA: U.S. Department of Health and Human Services.

De la TORRE, J. C. (2002). Vascular basis of Alzheimer's pathogenesis. *Annals of the New York Academy of Sciences, 977(1),* 196-215. doi: 10.1111/j.1749-6632.2002.tb04817.x

Dr. Fuhrman's Immunity Solution!. (2015). Retrieved from http://www.kpbs.org/news/2012/aug/07/dr-fuhrmans-immunity-solution/

Dr. McDougall's Health & Medical Center. (1970's). *The Lost Lectures from Nathan Pritikin.* Retrieved from https://www.drmcdougall.com/health/education/podcast/nathan-pritikin/

Greger, M., (2014). *How to prevent pre diabetes from turning into diabetes.* Retrieved from:

http://nutritionfacts.org/video/how-to-prevent-prediabetes-from-turning-into-diabetes

Harman, D. (1972). The biologic clock: the mitochondria?. *Journal of the American Geriatrics Society, 20(4),* 145-147. doi: 10.1111/j.1532-5415.1972.tb00787.x

Harnly, J. M., Doherty, R. F., Beecher, G. R., Holden, J. M., Haytowitz, D. B., Bhagwat, S., & Gebhardt, S. (2006). Flavonoid content of U.S. fruits, vegetables, and nuts. *J. Agric. Food Chem, 54(26).* 9966-9977. doi: 10.1021/jf061478a

Hyman MA. (2010). Environmental toxins, obesity, and diabetes: an emerging risk factor. *Alternative Therapies, 16(2),* 56-58. Retrieved from http://drhyman.com/downloads/Diabetes-and-Toxins.pdf

Kirsch, I. (2014). Antidepressants and the Placebo Effect. *Zeitschrift Fur Psychologie,* 222(3), 128–134. doi:10.1027/2151-2604/a000176

Kovacic, J.C., & Fuster V. (2012). Atherosclerotic risk factors, vascular cognitive impairment, and Alzheimer disease. *Mt Sinai J Med, 79(6),* 664-673. doi: 10.1002/msj.21347

Marcovecchio, M.L., & Chiarelli, F. (2012). The effects of Acute and chronic stress on diabetes control. *Sci Signal, 5(247).* doi: 10.1126/scisignal.2003508.

Marcovecchio, M.L., Lucantoni, M., & Chiarelli, F. (2011). Role of chronic and acute hyperglycemia in the development of diabetes complications. *Diabetes Technology & Therapeutics, 13(3),* 389-394. doi:10.1089/dia.2010.0146.

NA. (1977). Cardiogenic Dementia. *The Lancet, 309(8001),* 27 – 28. doi:10.1016/S0140-6736(77)91660-9

Radzevičienė, L., & Ostrauskas, R. (2012). Egg consumption and the risk of type 2 diabetes mellitus: a case–control study. *Public*

Health   Nutrition, 15(8),   1437–1441.   doi:
10.1017/S1368980012000614

Roberts, W. C. (2009). Evaluating lipid-lowering trials in the twenty-first century. *American Journal of Cardiology, 103(9),* 1325–1328. doi:10.1016/j.amjcard.2009.02.008

Sepehrnia, B., Kamboh, M. I., Adams-Campbell, L. L., Bunker, C. H., Nwankwo, M., Majumder, P. P., & Ferrell, R. E. (1989). Genetic studies of human apolipoproteins. X. The effect of the apolipoprotein E polymorphism on quantitative levels of lipoproteins in Nigerian blacks. *American Journal of Human Genetics, 45(4),* 586–591.

Sweeney J. S. (1927). Dietary factors that influence the dextrose tolerance test. *Arch   Intern   Med.* 40(6), 818-830. doi:10.1001/archinte.1927.00130120077005

The U.S. Food and Drug Administration (FDA). (2012). *FDA announces safety changes in labeling for some cholesterol-lowering   drugs.* Retrieved   from: http://www.fda.gov/NewsEvents/Newsroom/PressAnnouncem ents/ucm293623.htm

Sample 1. (2014). Diets high in meat, eggs and dairy could be as harmful to health as smoking Retrieved August 22, 2016, from https://www.theguardian.com/scienece/2014 mar/04/animal-protein-diets-smoking-meat-eggs-dairy

OTHER SOURCES

- The Bible Genesis Chapter 1 verses 29,30 Daniel 1 verses 8 through 16

- The Loss Lectures of Nathan Pritikin

- The Pritikin Promise

- Open Access

- Pub Med.govs

- New England Journal of Medicine

- Diabetic Care

- Newcastle college (Dr. Taylor)

- The American Diabetes Association

- Sarah Klein and Catherine Price type III diabetes May 2016 prevention magazine

- Cholesterol Reducing Strategy writer Jill Weisenberger RDN, CDE diabetic living

- Adventist Studies Loma Linda University

- American Association for Cancer Research

- American Institute for Cancer Research

- Journal of Biochemistry: Oxford Journals/Medicine & Health & Science & Mathematics

- Journal of Medical Biochemistry

- The British Medical Journal

- The Lancet

- The China Study

- The Telomere Effect by Elizabeth Blackburn, PhD Elissa Epel, PhD